NEUROSCIENCE RESEARCH PROGRESS

PATHOPHYSIOLOGY OF BRAIN-BODY INTERACTIONS IN ANEURYSMAL SUBARACHNOID HEMORRHAGE

NEUROSCIENCE RESEARCH PROGRESS

Additional books in this series can be found on Nova's website under the Series tab.

Additional e-books in this series can be found on Nova's website under the eBooks tab.

NEUROSCIENCE RESEARCH PROGRESS

PATHOPHYSIOLOGY OF BRAIN-BODY INTERACTIONS IN ANEURYSMAL SUBARACHNOID HEMORRHAGE

BENJAMIN W. Y. LO

EDITED BY:

HITOSHI FUKUDA, MASAOMI KOYANAGI,
BENEDICT BENG-TECK TAW, YUSUKE NISHIMURA,
AURORA W. M. LO, YEE-YIN A. WAN,
MATTHEW WAI-MAN LUI, HIDETOSHI KASUYA,
ADRIAN UPTON, AND MITCHELL A. H. LEVINE

nova biomedical
New York

Library of Congress Cataloging-in-Publication Data

Library of Congress Control Number: 2017956843
ISBN: 978-1-53612-716-4

Published by Nova Science Publishers, Inc. † New York

Contents

Preface vii

Acknowledgments ix

About the Author xi

About the Editors xiii

Section One Pathophysiologic Mechanisms in Aneurysmal Subarachnoid Hemorrhage and Central Autonomic Networks in the Brain-Body Interface **1**
Benjamin W. Y. Lo, Hitoshi Fukuda, Masaomi Koyanagi, Adrian Upton and Mitchell A. H. Levine

Section Two Systematic Review of Prognostic Factors in Aneurysmal Subarachnoid Hemorrhage **35**
Benjamin W. Y. Lo, Hitoshi Fukuda and Mitchell A. H. Levine

Section Three	Alterations in Brain-Body Interface in Aneurysmal Subarachnoid Hemorrhage – Comparative Regression Analyses in Two Cohorts *Benjamin W. Y. Lo, Hitoshi Fukuda, Masaomi Koyanagi, Adrian Upton and Mitchell A. H. Levine*	**61**
Section Four	Aneurysmal Subarachnoid Hemorrhage Prognostic Decision-Making Algorithms – Comparative Analyses in Two Cohorts *Benjamin W. Y. Lo, Hitoshi Fukuda, Masaomi Koyanagi, Adrian Upton and Mitchell A. H. Levine*	**89**
Section Five	The Brain-Body Interface in Aneurysmal Subarachnoid Hemorrhage – Exploratory Analyses Using Artificial Neural Networks *Benjamin W. Y. Lo, Hitoshi Fukuda, Masaomi Koyanagi, Benedict Taw, Matthew Wai-Man Lui, Hidetoshi Kasuya, Adrian Upton and Mitchell A. H. Levine*	**105**
Section Six	Conclusion *Benjamin W. Y. Lo*	**121**
Index		**127**

Preface

This monograph entitled "Pathophysiology of Brain-Body Interactions in Aneurysmal Subarachnoid Hemorrhage" is an up-to-date, in-depth and more advanced continuation of its accompanying monograph entitled "Brain-Body Interactions – Contemporary Outcome Prediction in Aneurysmal Subarachnoid Hemorrhage using Bayesian Neural Networks and Fuzzy Logic." The current monograph is divided into five sections. The first section synthesizes the most current evidence of underlying pathophysiologic mechanisms of brain-body associations in aneurysmal subarachnoid hemorrhage. It also describes pathophysiologic manifestations of central autonomic nervous system dysfunctions in ischemic stroke, intracerebral hemorrhage and aneurysmal subarachnoid hemorrhage. The second section synthesizes and critically appraises the methodologic quality of existing studies (including prospective and retrospective cohort studies and randomized controlled trials) that derive clinical predictor tools and clinical predictors used to determine outcome prognosis in patients with aneurysmal subarachnoid hemorrhage. The third section makes use of two aneurysmal subarachnoid hemorrhage databases incorporating advances in the treatment of aneurysmal subarachnoid hemorrhage. Both single prognostic factors and brain-body interactions are explored to make several novel observations which significantly influence clinical outcome in patients with ruptured cerebral aneurysms. In its fourth section, clinical prognostic decision-making tools are created using classification and regression tree analysis. Prognostic subgroups demonstrate the interplay of various underlying pathophysiologic mechanisms which, together, adversely influence long-term neurologic and functional outcomes in those with aneurysmal subarachnoid hemorrhage. Finally, in Section Five, exploratory analyses are conducted using artificial neural networks to further explore the brain-body interface in aneurysmal subarachnoid hemorrhage, with in-depth discussions of the autonomic nervous system and its dysfunction in pathologic states. Using these clinical prognostic models, the clinician can tailor individual-specific treatment efforts to prevent and treat various alterations in the brain-body interface in order to maximize the chances of survival and recovery after aneurysmal subarachnoid hemorrhage.

Acknowledgments

I would like to acknowledge Professors Mitchell Levine, Forough Farrohkyar and Lehana Thabane for their expertise in manuscript feedback and revision. The Tirilazad database was provided by Dr. Loch Macdonald. The Kurashiki Central Hospital database was provided by Dr. Hitoshi Fukuda. I would like to thank my family members who supported me during manuscript preparation. In addition, I would like to thank my current work colleagues at Montreal Neurological Institute and overseas in Hong Kong and Japan for their support.

About the Author

Benjamin W. Y. Lo, BSc MD MSc PhD FRCSC, is a cerebrovascular neurosurgeon and ICU specialist at Montreal Neurological Institute & Hospital, McGill University, Montreal, Canada. He is a current MNI Killam Scholar with graduate degrees (MSc, PhD) in clinical epidemiology and biostatistics. In his cerebrovascular neurosurgical operations and medical treatments of cerebrovascular patients in both the neurocritical care and stroke units, he applies his knowledge of brain-body interactions to make new clinical observations and treatment discoveries. His current languages include English, Chinese, French, Japanese and Spanish.

About the Editors

Hitoshi Fukuda, MD PhD, is a hybrid Japanese brain surgeon who does complex open cerebrovascular surgery as well as minimally invasive endovascular surgery in both adults and pediatrics. He and his colleagues at Kochi University and the Kyoto University system have developed significant advances in the diagnosis and treatment of aneurysmal subarachnoid hemorrhage. He has also provided valuable insights into the contents of this monograph.

Masaomi Koyanagi, MD PhD, is a hybrid Japanese brain surgeon who does minimally invasive endovascular surgery as well as open cerebrovascular surgery. He and his colleagues at the Kyoto University system have developed significant advances in the diagnosis and treatment of aneurysmal subarachnoid hemorrhage. He has also provided valuable insights into the contents of this monograph.

Benedict Beng-Teck Taw, MBBS(Adel), FRCSEd(SN), FHKAM(Surgery), is a functional neurosurgeon at Queen Mary Hospital, University of Hong Kong, Hong Kong. He provided feedback into the organization of this monograph as well as its translated version.

Yusuke Nishimura, MD PhD is the director of spine surgery at Nagoya University Hospital, Nagoya University, Japan.

Aurora W. M. Lo, BCom CPA, is a polyglot CPA (Illinois). She is also a freelance illustrator. She provided all illustrations and figures to this monograph. She has also provided valuable insights into the translated version of its accompanying monograph.

Yee-Yin A. Wan, BA MBA DBA, is an assistant professor in the Department of Business Administration at Hong Kong Shue Yan University. He has made a number of significant contributions to the fields of Management, Knowledge Management, Business Strategy, Business Anthropology and Marketing. Dr. Wan has provided valuable insights into the translated version of its accompanying monograph.

Matthew Wai-Man Lui, MBBS(HK), FRCSEd, FCSHK, FHKAM(Surgery) is a world renowned expert in cerebrovascular neurosurgery. He is the Chief of Neurosurgery and Consultant at Queen Mary Hospital, University of Hong Kong. He has provided valuable insights in this subject area.

Hidetoshi Kasuya, MD DMSc, is a world renowned expert in cerebrovascular, tumour and skull base neurosurgery. He is an expert in the areas of cerebral aneurysm, subarachnoid hemorrhage and vasospasm. Currently, Professor Kasuya is professor of neurosurgery at the Institute for Integrated Medical Sciences (TIIMS), Tokyo Women's Medical University, as well as visiting professor at Tokushima University, Japan. Professor Kasuya has over 150 peer-reviewed publications, 200 reviews, editorials and other related published papers. He has also provided valuable insights into the contents of this monograph.

Adrian Upton, MA MB BChir LRCP MRCS, is a world renowned neurologist, currently Professor Emeritus of the Division of Neurology, Department of Medicine, McMaster University. Dr. Upton completed his studies in Natural Sciences (1961) and Psychology (1962) at Cambridge University. He worked at Guy's Hospital, the London Chest Hospital, Whittington Hospital, Queen Square and Newcastle General Hospital, before becoming a long-term Chief of Neurology at McMaster University (since 1980) and Director of the Regional Epilepsy and Diagnostic Neurophysiology clinics (since 1971). Dr. Upton is an active pediatric and adult clinical neurologist and sees over 60 patients per week. He has over 410 publications, 130 peer-reviewed articles, co-author of 7 books and over 380 invited presentations around the world. He has also provided valuable insights into the contents of this monograph.

Mitchell A. H. Levine, BSc MSc MD FRCPC FISPE FACP, is the current Assistant Dean of the Department of Clinical Epidemiology & Biostatistics (Health Methods, Evidence and Impact) at McMaster University, Hamilton, Ontario, Canada. He is an internal medicine and clinical pharmacologist consultant, and is currently Professor in the department of Health Research Methods, Evidence and Impact, and the department of Medicine at McMaster University. Dr. Levine is the Director of the Centre for the Evaluation of Medicines, St. Joseph's Hospital. He has provided valuable insights and feedback into the contents of this monograph.

Section One

Pathophysiologic Mechanisms in Aneurysmal Subarachnoid Hemorrhage and Central Autonomic Networks in the Brain-Body Interface

***Benjamin W. Y. Lo*[1,*], *Hitoshi Fukuda*[2], *Masaomi Koyanagi*[3], *Adrian Upton*[4] and *Mitchell A. H. Levine*[5]**

[1]Departments of Neurosurgery,
Neurology and Critical Care Medicine,
Montreal Neurological Institute and Hospital,
McGill University, Montreal, Canada
[2]Department of Neurosurgery, Kochi University Hospital,
Kochi, Japan

---

[*] Corresponding Author Email: benjamin.lo@mcgill.ca.

[3]Department of Neurosurgery,
National Hospital Organization Himeji Medical Center,
Himeji, Japan
[4]Division of Neurology, Department of Medicine,
McMaster University, Hamilton, Ontario, Canada
[5]Department of Clinical Epidemiology & Biostatistics
(Department of Health Research Methods, Evidence and Impact),
Department of Medicine, Division of Clinical Pharmacology,
Centre for Evaluation of Medicines, St. Joseph's Hospital,
McMaster University, Hamilton, Ontario, Canada

Part One – Introduction to Aneurysmal Subarachnoid Hemorrhage

Defects in the medial layer or internal elastic lamina of an arterial wall lead to formation of a brain aneurysm. Cerebral aneurysms often form at blood vessels' branch or bifurcation points (Figure 1.1).

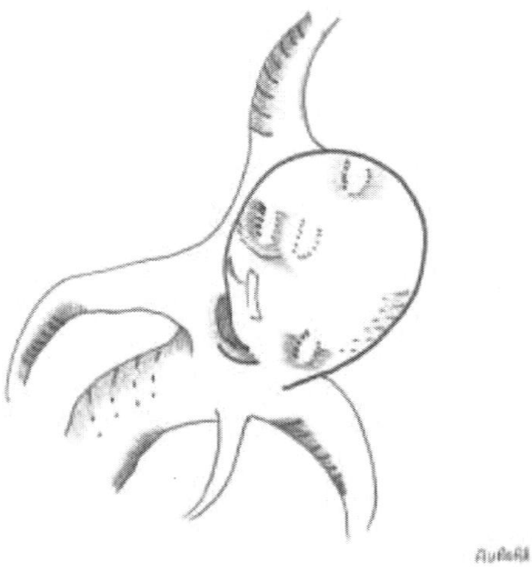

Figure 1.1. Cerebral aneurysm.

Pathologically, the combination of maldevelopment and degeneration may trigger the formation and rupture of an aneurysm. With wear and tear, hemodynamic stresses on the arterial bifurcation points may explain a higher incidence of ruptured aneurysms in those over the age of 60. Other than age, risk factors such as hypertension, smoking, obesity and arteriosclerosis also predispose aneurysms to rupture.

Aneurysmal rupture causes subarachnoid hemorrhage. Spontaneous subarachnoid hemorrhage is caused by aneurysmal rupture by 65% of cases. Other causes include:

1. rupture of other cerebral vascular malformations,
2. blood-related disorders (hematologic dyscrasias), such as malignancy, and
3. extension of blood clot in the brain (intracerebral hemorrhage) into the subarachnoid space.

Intracranial aneurysmal subarachnoid hemorrhage (SAH) affects about 45,000 individuals in North America and 600,000 individuals worldwide annually. Patients with ruptured brain aneurysms and aneurysmal subarachnoid hemorrhage have a mortality rate of at least 45% in the first month after rupture. Neurological damage can be from the primary injury of aneurysm rupture itself and a number of other secondary injurious processes that can further worsen the affected individual's neurological state. Figure 1.2 illustrates the spectrum of primary and secondary injuries after subarachnoid hemorrhage.

Explanations for each step are given below:

1. rupture of a brain aneurysm
2. increased intracranial pressure results in decreased blood flow to brain
3. brain swelling

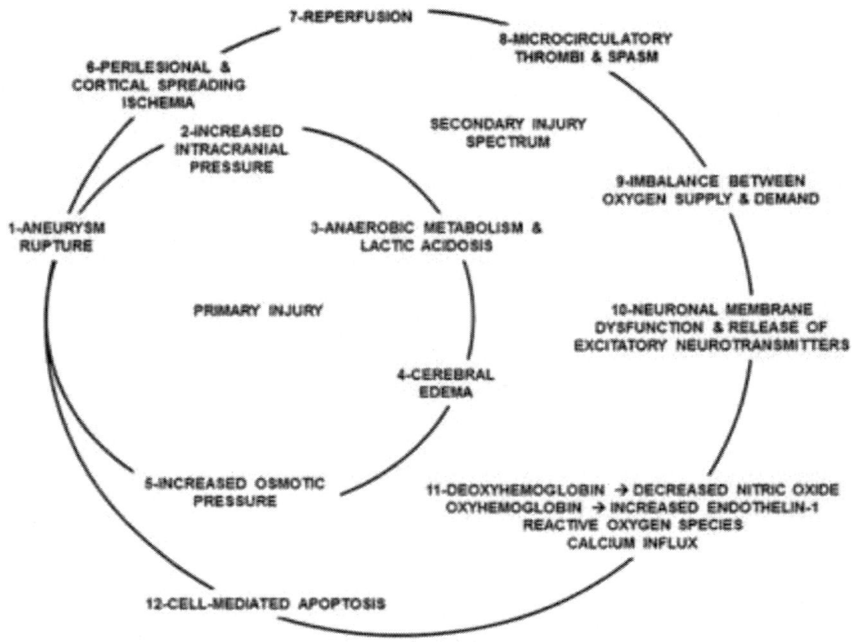

Figure 1.2. Spectrum of primary and secondary injuries after subarachnoid hemorrhage.

4. metabolism under lack of oxygen leading to formation and release of lactic acid
5. fluid leaks across disrupted blood-brain barrier
6. lack of blood flow and oxygen spread from site of aneurysm rupture to across the entire brain
7. injurious process when brain attempts to re-supply blood and oxygen to involved areas
8. clotting is triggered in small vessels, along with induced constriction of vessels of different sizes (vasospasm)
9. not enough oxygen is supplied via brain blood flow to meet the metabolic requirements of the damaged brain areas
10. nerve cell membranes are disrupted and further damage is caused with release of a number of chemicals that are toxic to the injured regions

11. products (including reactive oxygen species, endothelin-1, decreased nitric oxide, calcium) trigger deleterious processes (such as seizures, vasospasm, delayed strokes)
12. process of programmed cell death is triggered

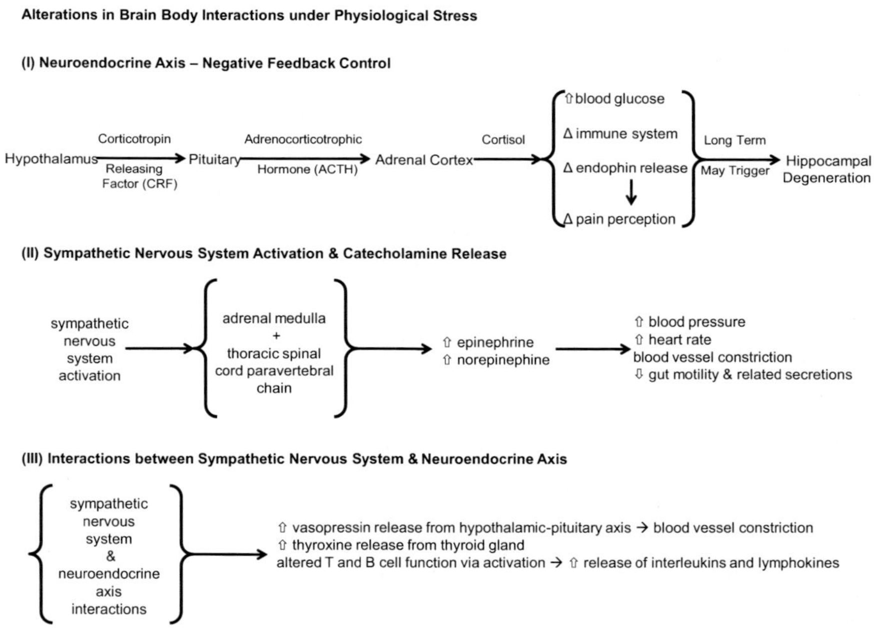

Figure 1.3. Demonstrates how brain-body interactions are altered under physiological stress.

Secondary injurious processes can be related to the nervous system such as re-bleeding from the ruptured aneurysm, brain swelling, occurrence of a delayed stroke, brain blood vessel vasospasm leading to seizures, delayed strokes and increase in brain-spinal fluid causing hydrocephalus. In addition, systemic medical complications are possible, such as myocardial infarction, fever and pulmonary edema. Together, these processes can lead to long-term disability. Types of disability include physical, neurocognitive and psychological impairment. Long-term reductions in health-related quality of life are common, even though the case fatality of aneurysmal SAH has slowly declined due to prompt diagnosis and repair, as well as improved critical care medical management. Figure 1.3 demonstrates how brain-body interactions are altered under physiological stress.

Part Two – The Brain-Body Interface and Autonomic Nervous System

The Brain-Body Interface and Autonomic Nervous System – Cardiovascular-Nervous System Associations

Direct and indirect projections of the autonomic nervous system control the cardiovascular system. These projects act via the parabrachial nucleus of the midbrain and pons (Figure 1.4). The parabrachial nucleus is a relay station that transmits signals between the cerebral cortex (especially limbic cortex), amygdala, hypothalamic paraventricular nucleus, vasomotor area of the lower brainstem (including the ventrolateral medulla, medullary raphe, nucleus of the solitary tract), and the thoracolumbar interomediolateral gray column of the spinal cord.

Autonomic visceral afferents from the thoracolumbar (sympathetic) and craniosacral (parasympathetic) levels ascend to the nucleus tractus solitarius. In addition, afferents from arterial baroreceptors in the aortic arch and carotid bodies also reach the nucleus tractus solitarius. This nucleus of the solitary tract also receives information about humoral (such as plasma electrolytes) and cerebrospinal chemical information from the area postrema (a circumventricular organ). Autonomic efferents include the anterior cingulate gyrus, amygdala, insula, hypothalamus, periaqueductal gray matter within the diencephalon, locus ceruleus, parabrachial nucleus of pons before final pathways within the medulla and intermediolateral spinal cord (Figure 1.5).

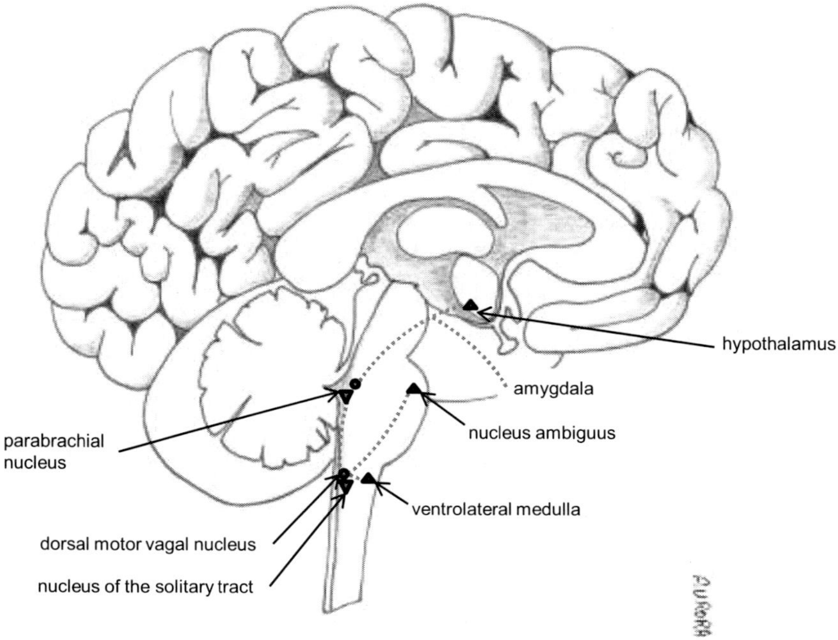

Figure 1.4. The central autonomic nervous system is excessively activated after brain aneurysm rupture.

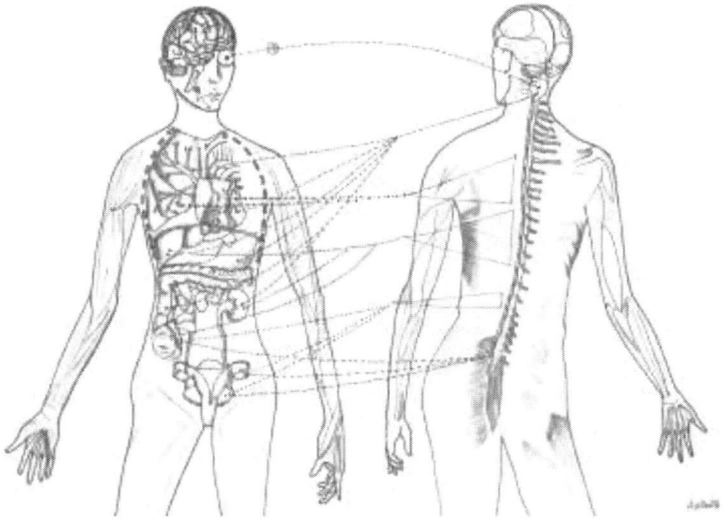

Figure 1.5. Shows the inter-relationships between the nervous system and other body organ systems.

Arterial baroceptors in the carotid sinus and aortic arch send information about arterial wall stretch to the nucleus tractus solitarius via the glossopharyngeal and vagus nerves. In so doing, the autonomic nervous system mediates the heart rate (chronotrophy), rate of nervous impulse transmission through the cardiac conductive tissue (dromotropy), and force of contraction (inotropy). Blood vessel diameter and tone are also mediated via the autonomic nervous system. Nucleus tractus solitarius inhibits the rostral ventrolateral medulla, excites the nucleus ambiguus and dorsal motor nucleus of vagus, producing a reduction in sympathetic tone and increase in vagal activity (including negative inotropic effects via the sinoatrial node as well as vasodilatory effects). Adrenergic neurons originating between T1 and L2 synapse with the entire arterial tree.

Counter-regulatory feedback with the sympathetic nervous system predominates. An example of such counter-regulatory feedback is the Cushing reflex. Increase in intracranial pressure from disease states, such as intracerebral hemorrhage, leads to decreased levels of oxygen and increased local levels of hydrogen ions and carbon dioxide around the vasomotor regions of the lower brainstem secondary to anaerobic metabolism. As a counter-regulatory measure, the systemic blood pressure is elevated in an attempt to increase blood flow to the brain. With this increase in blood pressure, heart rate is reflexively decreased via the arterial baroreceptors.

Other factors also affect the amount of autonomic nervous output from the vasomotor regions of the brainstem, including:

1. blood oxygen level,
2. blood carbon dioxide level,
3. pain stimulus,
4. chemoreceptors and baroreceptors in the carotid, pulmonary, and aortic vessels sense corresponding changes,

5. nerve impulse feedback from the lungs secondary to lung inflation and deflation, and
6. regulatory signals between the cerebral cortex and brainstem.

Heart rate variability can reflect the balance of sympathetic and parasympathetic nervous activity. The QRS complex's RR interval time series reflect heart rate variability, sensing changes in atrioventricular conduction affecting cardiac output and stroke volume. Low frequency power (0.05-0.15 Hz) of heart rate variability is under the combined influence of sympathetic and parasympathetic tones, with sympathetic modulation by the sinus node. Increases in low frequency power represent decreased vagal activity. High frequency power (0.15-0.4 Hz) of heart rate variability reflects parasympathetic modulation of cardiac activity, a measure which is influenced by respirations. In respiratory sinus arrthymias, heart rate oscillations are caused by ventilation with slight heart rate increases with each inspiratory cycle due to transient decreases in parasympathetic tone. Therefore, the high frequency to low frequency ratio can be regarded as a measure of sympathovagal balance.

As illustrated, the autonomic nervous system adjusts blood pressures by adjusting heart rate, cardiac contractility and peripheral vascular resistance, where the baroreceptors measure blood pressures by sensing blood vessel stretch located in the aorta, carotid arteries and large veins. Baroreceptor activity sends afferent activity to regulate blood pressure through: (1) baroreflex – with systolic blood pressures as inputs and RR interval changes as outputs through the sinoatrial node, and (2) sympathetic vasomotor tone – with diastolic blood pressures as inputs and outputs through muscle sympathetic nervous activity to control blood vessel constriction and peripheral vascular resistance. Baroreceptor sensitivity reflects the capability of the baroreflex to adjust heart rates to changing conditions. The baroreceptor sensitivity can be regarded as the ratio of heart rate changes in response to fixed changes in blood pressures.

The Brain-Body Interface – Respiratory-Nervous System Associations

Pacemaker cells in the medulla are responsible for the autonomic control of respiration. Their rhythmic discharges are modified by pneumotaxic neurons in the pons, as well as limbic and hypothalamic lesions. Other contributions include:

1. impulses from afferent pulmonary vagal fibers with lung inflation and deflation,
2. spinal reflexes from cervical and thoracic spinal cord to the diaphragm and intercostal muscles,
3. changes in the cerebrospinal fluid concentrations of carbon dioxide and hydrogen ions sensed by medullary chemoreceptors, and
4. changes in oxygen tension sensed by baroreceptors in the aorta, cardiac atrium, and ventricle, as well as pulmonary arteries.

The Brain-Body Interface –Endocrinological-Nervous System Associations

The hypothalamic-pituitary axis regulates the key aspects of homeostasis, temperature control, and endocrinological functions. This system integrates inputs from both the limbic system and brainstem in order to modulate both emotional and instinctual reactions to changes in the internal milieu.

The Brain-Body Interface –Gastrointestinal-Nervous System Associations

The gastrointestinal autonomic nervous system regulates the central nervous system inputs to the enteric system regarding gut motility and secretory functions. It works in conjunction with local paracrine pathways.

Part Three – Evidence Assessment of Pathophysiologic Mechanisms of Brain-Body Associations in Aneurysmal Subarachnoid Hemorrhage

Current evidence in the pathophysiologic mechanisms of brain-body associations in aneurysmal subarachnoid hemorrhage is illustrated with six articles.

Study Eligibility Criteria

Studies that were eligible for this evidence systematic review included:

1. studies of adult patients with ruptured brain aneurysms,
2. these patients received diagnostic tests to investigate pathophysiologic mechanisms of brain-body associations in aneurysmal SAH,
3. these patients also received reference standard investigations to document multi-organ deteriorations after brain aneurysm rupture, and
4. prospective and retrospective cohort studies and randomized controlled trials investigating pathophysiologic mechanisms of brain-body associations in aneurysmal SAH.

We excluded the following studies:

1. those that do not characterize pathophysiologic mechanisms of brain-body associations,
2. those that do not distinguish between aneurysmal and non-aneurysmal SAH, and
3. studies based on expert opinions.

Eligible studies were limited to those published from January 1, 2000 to March 31, 2014. We truncated eligible studies to this time period because of advancements in:

1. investigations to diagnose aneurysmal SAH, such as computed tomography (CT) angiogram,
2. diagnostic tests to investigate pathophysiologic mechanisms of brain-body associations, such as advanced pulse contour analysis for cardiopulmonary parameters and blood assays for neuroendocrine markers, and
3. surgical and neurocritical care treatment differences such as availability of minimally invasive endovascular techniques.

Literature Search

Two reviewers (Benjamin Lo [BL], Hitoshi Fukuda [HF]) independently searched a number of electronic databases. Relevant studies were identified from Ovid MEDLINE, Ovid EMBASE, Web of Science, the Cumulative Index to Nursing and Allied Health Literature, without language restrictions. To include gray literature, we also searched ProceedingsFirst and PapersFirst. We used the search terms:

1. "aneurysmal subarachnoid hemorrhage" and "cardio-pulmonary,"
2. "aneurysmal subarachnoid hemorrhage" and "renal,"

3. "aneurysmal subarachnoid hemorrhage" and "gastrointestinal,"
4. "aneurysmal subarachnoid hemorrhage" and "immune" and "hematologic," and
5. "aneurysmal subarachnoid hemorrhage" and "brain-body associations."

Study Selection and Data Collection Process

Both investigators (BL and HF) reviewed all titles and abstracts, and full reports of all potentially relevant trials. The initial literature search (January 1, 2000 – March 31, 2014) yielded 150 citations (Figure 2). Screening by title and abstract and citation yielded 88 items. Of these 88 items, reviewers BL and HF reached agreement on 41 items for inclusion, 38 items for exclusion and were unsure on 9 items. Interrater reliability was high (estimated kappa 0.81 (95% CI 0.76-0.87) for citation and abstract screening). Fifty full text articles were identified as potentially relevant, and were assessed, with further exclusion of articles due to:

1. inappropriate patient inclusion and exclusion criteria,
2. inadequate outcome reporting, and
3. discussions lacking pathophysiologic mechanisms of brain-body associations in aneurysmal SAH.

Investigators BL and HF then independently applied the inclusion criteria to the full reports. Each trial report was examined carefully for its methodologic quality. As outlined in the "methodologic quality assessment" section, each article was appraised in nine areas. Of the 54 items assessed in six articles, BL and HF reached agreement on 43 items, disagreed on 8 items and were unsure on 3 items (kappa statistic = 0.82, 95% CI 0.71-0.93). For data collection, the reviewers

(BL, HF) extracted relevant data using a data extraction form, piloted on a sample of included studies.

Assessment of Pathophysiologic Mechanisms of Brain-Body Associations in Aneurysmal Subarachnoid Hemorrhage

For this systematic review, the following items were reviewed in order to clarify pathophysiologic mechanisms of brain-body associations in aneurysmal SAH:

1. study design – including description of study protocol, study setting and recruitment,
2. patient population – including representativeness of cohort, inclusion and exclusion criteria, and sample size,
3. investigations – including reference tests to document organ dysfunction and diagnostic tests to document how ruptured brain aneurysms affect other organs,
4. outcome – including discussions on pathophysiologic mechanisms of brain-body associations in aneurysmal SAH, and
5. ethical conduct of study – including institutional ethics board approval and funding declarations.

Methodologic Quality Assessment

For this systematic review, we sampled the QUADAS-2 tool (Quality Assessment of Diagnostic Accuracy Studies Tool – Revised Version. The following areas were used in methodologic quality assessment as they would apply to pathophysiologic mechanisms of brain-body associations in aneurysmal SAH:

1. whether subjects included are representative of those treated in clinical practice,
2. clear study designs and descriptions of study protocols, inclusion and exclusion criteria, study settings and recruitment,
3. inclusion of study findings with adequate discussions of pathophysiologic mechanisms of brain-body associations in aneurysmal SAH,
4. clear descriptions of reference standards to document multi-organ dysfunction,
5. whether diagnostic tests to investigate brain-body associations were described in sufficient detail to permit test replication,
6. whether clinical data for study subjects are reproducible for those treated in clinical practice,
7. reporting of non-interpretable test results,
8. explanation of study withdrawals, and
9. whether the measure is clinically useful.

Study Search and Selection

The initial literature search (January 1, 2000 – March 31, 2014) yielded 150 citations (Figure 1.6). These were screened by title and abstract. Fifty full text articles were identified as potentially relevant, and were assessed, with further exclusion of articles due to inappropriate patient inclusion and exclusion criteria, inadequate outcome reporting, and discussions lacking pathophysiologic mechanisms of brain-body associations in aneurysmal SAH. Six studies were included in this systematic review. A meta-analysis was not feasible in this review to statistically pool outcomes obtained from the included studies clarifying pathophysiologic mechanisms of brain-body associations in ruptured brain aneurysms. Marked between-study differences were noted in the included studies with: (1) differing diagnostic tests and reference value ranges, (2) differing clinical outcome endpoint measures, and (3) scarcity of studies investigating each type of diagnostic investigation.

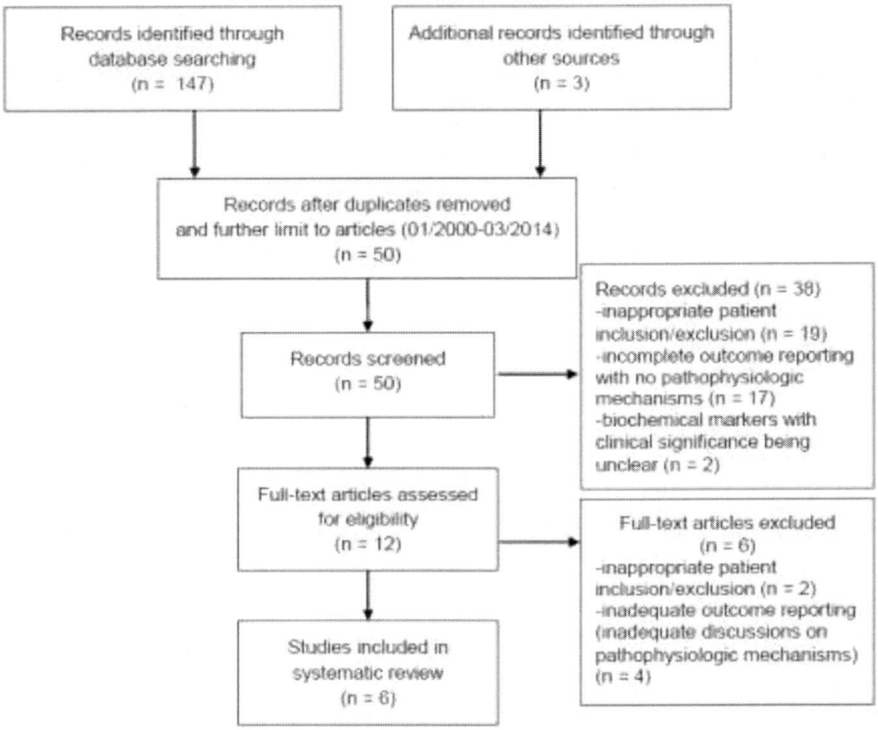

Figure 1.6. Flow diagram of study selection.

Diagnostic tests of serum and cerebrospinal fluid markers were studied in four out of six studies, radiographic investigations in two out of six studies, and invasive pulmonary artery thermodilution parameters in two out of six studies. In addition, there is no standardization of diagnostic tests between investigating centers.

Study Results and Synthesis of Results

This systematic review identified five prospective cohort studies and one retrospective study for inclusion in the analysis. Of the six methodologically rigorous studies identified for this systematic review, pathophysiologic mechanisms were clarified between the brain and the following organ systems:

1. cardiac system – six out of six studies,
2. pulmonary system – three out of six studies,
3. endocrine system – three out of six studies,
4. renal system (including electrolyte and fluid balance) – three out of six studies,
5. immune and hematologic systems – zero studies, and
6. gastrointestinal system – zero studies.

Assessment of Pathophysiologic Mechanisms of Brain-Body Associations in Aneurysmal Subarachnoid Hemorrhage for Included Studies

Article 1: Endocrine Response after Severe Subarachnoid Hemorrhage Related To Sodium and Blood Volume Regulation

(Audibert G, Steinmann G, de Talancé, et al. Endocrine responses after severe subarachnoid hemorrhage related to sodium and blood volume regulation. Neurosurgical Anesthesiology and Neuroscience. 2009 June; 108(6);1922-1928.)

In this prospective cohort study, Audibert et al. investigated endocrinologic responses, as well as sodium and water regulation after severe aneurysmal SAH. Over a period of 2 years, 19 adults with aneurysmal SAH were included (average 47 years old). Totally, 12 patients were excluded because of the history of renal insufficiency, cardiac disease, chronic treatment with diuretics, angiotensin-converting enzyme inhibitors and steroids. Clear study protocols were described with the maintenance of euvolemia and sodium balance.

Reference standard tests that documented multi-organ involvement included an electrocardiogram, cardiac enzymes, echocardiography and transcranial Doppler ultrasound. Diagnostic tests performed to clarify brain-body associations included daily sodium excretion fraction, glomerular filtration rate, creatinine clearance, plasma levels of brain natriuretic peptide, atrial natriuretic peptide, aldosterone, renin, angiotensin II and vasopressin. This study found the following:

1. with maintenance of euvolemia and salt balance, only 1 out of 19 patients experienced severe clinical vasospasm,
2. levels of brain natriuretic peptide increased between days 1 and 3 after aneurysmal rupture,
3. levels of atrial natriuretic peptide increased between days 4 and 6 after aneurysmal rupture, with associated increases in levels of renin, aldosterone and angiotensin II, and
4. levels of vasopressin increased between days 10 and 12 after aneurysmal rupture.

This study clearly describes the relationship between brain aneurysmal rupture and delayed activation of renin-angiotensin-aldosterone system. It had institutional ethics board approval, and clear declaration of funding sources. However, its main weaknesses included small study sample size, patient selection and center referral biases.

Article 2: Neuro-Cardio-Endocrine Response to Acute Subarachnoid Hemorrhage

(Espiner E, Leikis R, Ferch R, et al. The neuro-cardio-endocrine response to acute subarachnoid hemorrhage. Clinical Endocrinology. 2002; 56:629-635.)

In this prospective cohort study, Espiner et al. investigated relationships between neurologic, cardiac and endocrine responses after severe aneurysmal SAH. Over a period of 2 years, 18 adults with aneurysmal SAH were included (average 54 years old). Exclusion criteria included history of renal, hepatic, cardiac, endocrine diseases and history of diuretic and angiotensin converting enzyme inhibitor use prior to hospitalization. Clear study protocols were described. Patients were prescribed tapering doses of dexamethasone on admission. Reference standard tests that documented multi-organ involvement included an electrocardiogram, cardiac enzymes, chest radiographs. Diagnostic tests performed to clarify brain-body associations included plasma levels of cardiac enzymes, endothelin, brain natriuretic peptide and atrial natriuretic peptide, cerebrospinal fluid levels of brain natriuretic peptide, and atrial natriuretic peptide. This study found the following:

1. Brain natriuretic peptide and atrial natriuretic peptide levels in plasma increased in the first 3 days post-aneurysmal rupture. They returned to normal levels by day 7. Cerebrospinal fluid levels of brain natriuretic peptide and atrial natriuretic peptide did not show any changes. Abnormal electrocardiograms were noted in 6 out of 7 patients.
2. Urinary sodium levels increased within the first 3 days then remained stable. Plasma sodium levels gradually decreased.
3. Plasma vasopressin levels were increased on presentation then fell to normal levels after 2 days. Plasma aldosterone and renin levels increased at day 10-12. Cortisol levels fell abruptly on day 3 and maintained low levels to day 10.
4. Initial elevations of epinephrine, norepinephrine and endothelin fell by day 3 and remained at subnormal levels.

This study thoroughly describes the various relationships between the brain, neuroendocrine and renal systems. It had institutional ethics board approval and clear declaration of funding sources. However, its main weakness is the treatment of patients with admission dose of dexamethasone which further delayed activation of the renin-angiotensin-aldosterone system. Patients also demonstrated depressed adrenal-hypothalamic cortisol axis. This study also had small study sample size. Other weaknesses included patient selection and center referral biases.

Article 3: Subarachnoid Hemorrhage Complicated with Neurogenic Pulmonary Edema and Tako-Tsubo-Like Cardiomyopathy

(Inamasu J, Nakatsukasa M, Mayanagi K, et al. Subarachnoid hemorrhage complicated with neurogenic pulmonary edema and Tako-tsubo-like cardiomyopathy. Neurol Med Chir (Tokyo). 2012; 52:49-55.)

In this retrospective cohort study, Inamasu et al. characterized cardiopulmonary dysfunctions in aneurysmal SAH. Over a period of 5 years, 16 adults with aneurysmal SAH and neurogenic pulmonary edema were included (average 63 years). Exclusion criteria included patients with non-aneurysmal SAH. Clear study protocols were described. Patients were maintained euvolemic and had spinal catheters for clot clearance. Reference standard tests included electrocardiogram and chest radiograph. Diagnostic tests included a transthoracic echocardiogram. This study found the following:

1. Of 16 patients with neurogenic pulmonary edema, 14 had Tako-tsubo-like cardiomyopathy. All exhibited electrocardiographic changes (including ST segment abnormalities, QT prolongation and T-wave inversions). They were all intubated and were on vasopressors.
2. Neurogenic pulmonary edema was significantly associated with posterior circulation aneurysms ($p = 0.004$). 9 out of 16 patients died (7 from the primary aneurysmal rupture, 1 from rebleeding and 1 from vasospasm-induced strokes).

This study clearly demonstrated relationships between neurogenic pulmonary edema and Tako-tsubo-like cardiomyopathy. It had institutional ethics board approval and clear declaration of funding sources. However, its main weaknesses included small study sample size, patient selection and center referral biases.

Article 4: Cardiac Troponin Elevation, Cardiovascular Morbidity and Outcome after Subarachnoid Hemorrhage

(Naidech A, Kreiter K, Janjua N, et al. Cardiac troponin elevation, cardiovascular morbidity and outcome after subarachnoid hemorrhage. Circulation. 2005; 112:2851-2856.)

In this retrospective cohort study, Naidech et al. investigated relationships between cardiac troponin rise after aneurysmal SAH and its association with cardiopulmonary complications, delayed cerebral ischemia and death. Over a period of 4 years, 253 patients with SAH and electrocardiographic abnormalities were included (average 55 years). Exclusion criteria included patients with traumatic SAH and hemorrhage from arteriovenous malformations. Clear study protocols were described. Patients were maintained euvolemic. Reference standard tests included an electrocardiogram. Diagnostic tests included cardiac enzymes and chest radiographs. This study found the following:

1. Cardiac enzyme elevation was noted in patients who were older (average age 55 years), worse admission neurologic status, more blood on CT scan on admission, more physiologic dysfunction and hypertensive therapy.
2. Cardiac enzyme elevation was associated with risk of hypotension requiring vasopressors, left ventricular systolic dysfunction on echocardiogram, delayed cerebral ischemia from vasospasm and death.

This study demonstrated associations between cardiac troponin elevation and cardiovascular-related morbidity and mortality after aneurysmal SAH. It had institutional ethics board approval and clear declaration of funding sources. However, this study did not distinguish between aneurysmal and non-aneurysmal SAH. Furthermore, it did not discuss pathophysiologic mechanisms of brain-body associations in detail.

Article 5: Clinical Significance of Elevated Natriuretic Peptide Levels and Cardiopulmonary Parameters after Subarachnoid Hemorrhage

(Nakamura T, Okuchi K, Matsuyama T, et al. Clinical significance of elevated natriuretic peptide levels and cardiopulmonary parameters after subarachnoid hemorrhage. Neurol Med Chir (Tokyo). 2009; 49:185-192.)

In this prospective cohort study, Nakamura et al. investigated the relationships between natriuretic peptides and changes in cardiopulmonary parameters. Over a period of 2 years, 20 adults with aneurysmal SAH were included (average 65 years). Exclusion criteria included patients with a history of acute myocardial infarction, arrhythmia and congestive heart failure. Clear study protocols were described. Patients were maintained euvolemic. Reference standard tests included electrocardiograph, chest radiograph, echocardiograph and transcranial Doppler. Diagnostic tests included plasma levels of atrial natriuretic peptide and brain natriuretic peptide and pulse contour analysis to measure cardiopulmonary parameters. This PiCCO system measured cardiac index, systemic vascular resistance index, intrathoracic blood volume index and extravascular lung water index. This study found the following:

1. Plasma levels of brain natriuretic peptides peaked on post-aneurysm rupture day 1. Plasma levels of atrial natriuretic

peptide peaked on post-aneurysm rupture day 2, and remained increased up to day 6.
2. Natriuretic peptides caused sodium and water loss with plasma sodium levels falling between days 3 and 10.
3. There were no changes in cardiac indices and slight increases in extravascular lung water indices. There were no changes in intrathoracic blood volume indices.

This study thoroughly discussed relationships between elevated natriuretic peptides and cardiopulmonary parameters after aneurysmal SAH. It had institutional ethics board approval and clear declaration of funding sources. However, its main weaknesses included small study sample size, patient selection and center referral biases.

Article 6: Circulatory Characteristics of Normovolemia and Normotension Therapy after Subarachnoid Hemorrhage, Focusing on Pulmonary Edema

(Sato Y, Isotani E, Kubota Y, et al. Circulatory characteristics of normovolemia and normotension therapy after subarachnoid hemorrhage, focusing on pulmonary edema. Acta Neurochir. 2012; 154:2195-2202.)

In this prospective cohort study, Sato et al. characterized circulatory parameters after several aneurysmal SAH to reveal mechanisms of pulmonary edema. Over a period of 2 years, 49 adults with aneurysmal SAH were included (average 59 years). Exclusion criteria included patients with brainstem dysfunction and lack of study consent. Clear study protocols were described. Patients were maintained euvolemic. Reference standard tests included chest radiograph and arterial blood gases. Diagnostic tests included pulse contour analysis to measure cardiopulmonary parameters. This study found the following:

1. 7 out of 49 patients experienced neurogenic pulmonary edema.

2. Patients with neurogenic pulmonary edema had a lower cardiac function index and lower global ejection fraction. They had higher global end diastolic volume index.
3. Even though neurogenic pulmonary edema patients had net negative water balance and low central venous pressures, they had higher extravascular lung water index.

This study thoroughly discussed circulatory changes in aneurysmal SAH patients with neurogenic pulmonary edema. It had institutional ethics board approval, and clear declaration of funding sources. However, its main weaknesses included small study sample size, patient selection, and center selection biases.

Methodological Quality of Included Studies

In summary, all six studies have strong methodologic quality (Table 1.1). They had representative patient populations, clear selection criteria and clear descriptions of study designs. Reproducible study protocols with ethics board approval were present. Clinical results were described in sufficient detail and were applicable to aneurysmal SAH patients in clinical practice. There were few study withdrawals. These cases were medical deteriorations and deaths precluding study completion. The main methodologic weakness in all studies included small sample size, patient selection and center referral biases.

Results gained from these studies are clinically useful and shed light on how ruptured brain aneurysms affect the cardiopulmonary system. Subsequent neuro-cardio-endocrine responses then interact with other body systems, including the renal system, as part of the secondary responses to primary injury.

Table 1.1. Methodological assessment of articles on brain-body associations in aneurysmal subarachnoid hemorrhage

Study design	Audibert et al.	Espiner et al.	Inamasu et al.	Naidech et al.	Nakamura et al.	Sato et al.
	Prospective cohort	Prospective cohort	Prospective cohort	Retrospective cohort	Prospective cohort	Prospective cohort
Representativeness of cohort	Yes	Yes	Yes	Yes	Yes	Yes
Selection criteria	Clear	Clear	Clear	Clear	Clear	Clear
Reference standard used?	Yes	Yes	Yes	Yes	Yes	Yes
Index test reproducible?	Yes	Yes	Yes	Yes	Yes	Yes
Clinical data applicable to clinical practice?	Yes	Yes	Yes	Yes	Yes	Yes
Non-interpretable test results reported?	Yes	Yes	Yes	Yes	Yes	Yes
Withdrawals explained?	Yes	Yes	Yes	No study withdrawals	Yes	No study withdrawals
Measure clinically useful?	Yes	Yes	Yes	Yes	Yes	Yes

Part Four – The Brain-Body Interface in Aneurysmal Subarachnoid Hemorrhage

Brain-Heart Interactions in Aneurysmal Subarachnoid Hemorrhage

Rupture of brain aneurysms can lead to overactivity of the sympathetic nervous system. This triggers a sympathetic surge of catecholamine release from the thoracic spinal cord's paravertebral chain. Pathologically, the cardiac ventricle is stunned. This manifests as electrographic changes and troponin elevations. Troponin changes are more commonly found in those with poor neurological grade, intraventricular hemorrhage, cerebral edema, loss of consciousness at ictus, and multisystem physiological derangements. They are associated with adverse events including left ventricular systolic dysfunction, pulmonary edema, hypotension requiring vasopressors, delayed strokes, and death. Troponin release, however, are not usually as high as levels observed after myocardial infarction secondary to lack of coronary blood flow. Indeed, cardiac stunning refers to cardiac beta receptor hyperactivation and hypercontraction where contraction band necrosis can result. An extreme case of this, is the observation of stunned apical and mid-ventricular segments in takotsubo-like cardiomyopathy.

Electrocardiographic, troponin, and echocardiographic evidence correlate with blood measurement of brain natriuretic peptide, a protein released from the cardiac ventricle with peak values on post-rupture day 1. The brain site of brain natriuretic peptide production does not seem to be as affected as cerebrospinal fluid levels of brain natriuretic peptide are not elevated. Further physiologic evidence from pulse contour analysis points to a global decrease in cardiac ejection fraction, with a subsequent increase in extravascular lung water index by post-rupture day 3. This is consistent with increased catecholamines in peripheral arterioles which can increase pulmonary venous pressures and enhance pulmonary vascular permeability. The combination of increase pulmonary vascular permeability, increased pulmonary vascular pressure, decreased cardiac contractility, and increased volume from resuscitation can lead to hydrostatic pulmonary edema where hydrostatic pressures favoring edema formation overwhelms the opposing oncotic pressures. As a result of the apparent increased preload, the cardiac atrium is stretched. Plasma atrial natriuretic peptide levels peak at post-rupture day 2 after aneurysmal rupture. Cerebrospinal fluid levels of atrial natriuretic peptides remain normal suggesting that the primary source of atrial natriuretic peptide release is the cardiac atrium and not the brain.

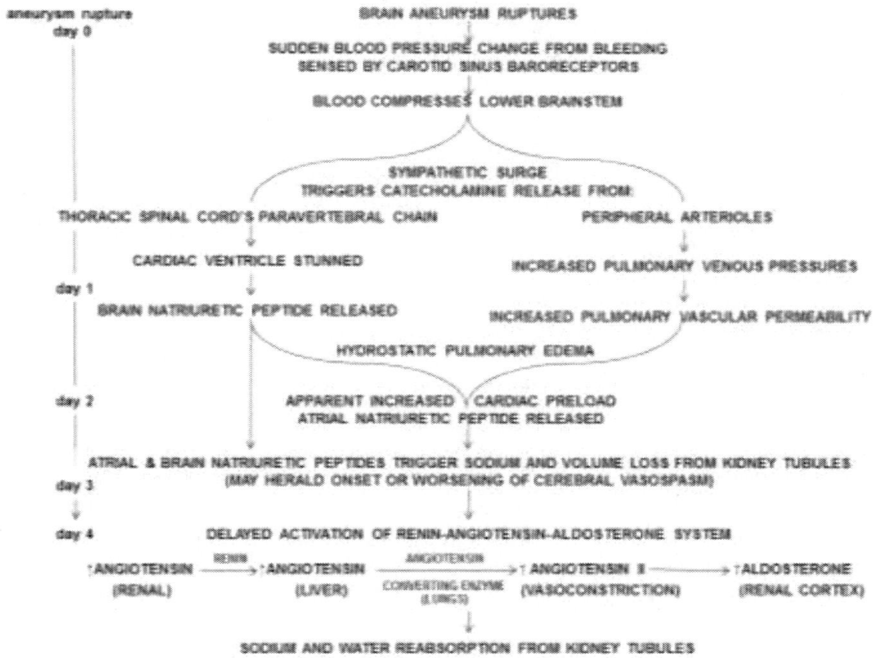
aneurysm rupture
day 0
BRAIN ANEURYSM RUPTURES
SUDDEN BLOOD PRESSURE CHANGE FROM BLEEDING
SENSED BY CAROTID SINUS BARORECEPTORS
BLOOD COMPRESSES LOWER BRAINSTEM
SYMPATHETIC SURGE
TRIGGERS CATECHOLAMINE RELEASE FROM
THORACIC SPINAL CORD'S PARAVERTEBRAL CHAIN
PERIPHERAL ARTERIOLES
CARDIAC VENTRICLE STUNNED
INCREASED PULMONARY VENOUS PRESSURES
day 1
BRAIN NATRIURETIC PEPTIDE RELEASED
INCREASED PULMONARY VASCULAR PERMEABILITY
HYDROSTATIC PULMONARY EDEMA
day 2
APPARENT INCREASED CARDIAC PRELOAD
ATRIAL NATRIURETIC PEPTIDE RELEASED
ATRIAL & BRAIN NATRIURETIC PEPTIDES TRIGGER SODIUM AND VOLUME LOSS FROM KIDNEY TUBULES
(MAY HERALD ONSET OR WORSENING OF CEREBRAL VASOSPASM)
day 3
day 4
DELAYED ACTIVATION OF RENIN-ANGIOTENSIN-ALDOSTERONE SYSTEM
↑ANGIOTENSIN
(RENAL)
↑ANGIOTENSIN
(LIVER)
↑ANGIOTENSIN II
(VASOCONSTRICTION)
↑ALDOSTERONE
(RENAL CORTEX)
SODIUM AND WATER REABSORPTION FROM KIDNEY TUBULES

Figure 1.7. Illustrates pathophysiologic mechanisms of brain-body associations after aneurysmal subarachnoid hemorrhage and delayed activation of the renin-angiotensin-aldosterone system.

Together, atrial and brain natriuretic peptides then act on renal tubules triggering sodium and volume loss. Without appropriate resuscitation, plasma sodium levels can fall drastically by post-rupture day 4–6. This drop can be attenuated with preemptive judicious volume and salt replacement. With this treatment, the incidence of severe clinical vasospasm can be lowered. Natriuretic and diuretic states in aneurysmal subarachnoid hemorrhage often herald the onset of clinical vasospasm. Between days 4 and 6, the renin-angiotensin-aldosterone system is activated. Figure 1.7 shows pathophysiologic mechanisms of brain-body associations after aneurysmal subarachnoid hemorrhage, as well as interrelationships, between the neuro-cardio-endocrine systems and the renin-angiotensin-aldosterone system. This system is activated in a delayed manner as a compensatory mechanism for prior sodium and water loss. Waiting for this mechanism alone to compensate for sodium and water balance in the aneurysmal subarachnoid hemorrhage patient will have severe negative consequences because the onset of vasospasm can lead to delayed strokes and further secondary neurological damage.

Brain-Lung Interactions in Aneurysmal Subarachnoid Hemorrhage

In addition to cardiac changes, cardiopulmonary and pulmonary changes occur after brain aneurysm rupture. Early after aneurysmal subarachnoid hemorrhage, cardiopulmonary changes are observed. With brain aneurysm rupture, massive catecholamine surges increase blood pressure in the pulmonary vessels (both arteries and veins) leading to pulmonary hypertension. Catecholamine surges also directly damage blood vessel endothelium. This creates a leaky pulmonary vasculature. Pulmonary edema can occur if:

1. the heart is concurrently stunned and cannot pump properly resulting in increased preload, and
2. pulmonary hypertension exists and is transmitted to the pulmonary capillaries increasing the pulmonary capillary pressure.

In aneurysmal subarachnoid hemorrhage, hydrostatic pulmonary edema occurs. Here, the amount of hydrostatic pressure (outward pressure favouring fluid to leak across pulmonary vessels from increases pressure, vasodilation and increased preload) is greater than the amount of oncotic pressure (tendency of fluid to stay within blood vessels because of proteins in blood keeping fluids there). This illustrates the concept of altered Starling forces.

In later stages after aneurysmal subarachnoid hemorrhage, patients are also susceptible to:

1. pneumonia (lung infections because of decreased cough mechanisms, compromised immune systems and retained oral secretions, including those pooling around ventilator breathing tubes), and
2. pulmonary embolism – immobility and systemic inflammatory states can predispose to formation of deep venous thrombosis with subsequent breakage of clots which can travel to pulmonary vessels.

Other Brain-Body Interactions in Aneurysmal Subarachnoid Hemorrhage

Other types of brain-body interactions observed after aneurysmal subarachnoid hemorrhage include:

1. hyperglycermia – this metabolic change can lower neuronal ischemic threshold and lead to larger stroke volumes. It can also lead to altered endothelial function, increased free radical production and inflammatory cell migration.
2. anemia – this change decreases the blood's oxygen carrying capacity can increase neuronal hypoxic damage and stroke volumes.
3. altered sodium levels as a reflection of altered kidney function and neurohumoral activation (including cortisol, natriuretic peptides, vasopressin and catecholamines). Sodium level alterations and disrupted blood brain barriers can lead to cerebral edema.
4. systemic inflammatory states after brain aneurysm rupture can lead to derangements in coagulation with abnormalities in both thrombosis and fibrinolysis. Higher levels of fibrinolytic markers, along with inflammatory cytokines, are seen after aneurysmal subarachnoid hemorrhage.
5. altered gastrointestinal motility after aneurysmal subarachnoid hemorrhage with initial phase of accelerated gastric emptying followed by late phase of decreased intestinal motility. Hypercatabolic states (at least 25 kcal/kg/day) are also observed with increased nitrogen loss. Patients are also at higher risk of gastric ulcers.
6. occurrence of fevers after brain aneurysms can markedly increase cerebral metabolic rates. This can herald delayed strokes, and worsen ischemic injury and cerebral edema. Early onset fevers are more likely to be due to central (hypothalamic) damage. Late onset fevers are more likely to be due to infections, but can include fevers secondary to pulmonary embolism and drug-drug interactions.

Conclusion

This section synthesizes the most current evidence of underlying pathophysiologic mechanisms of brain related associations with body systems in aneurysmal SAH. It also summarizes manifestations of central autonomic network dysfunction in aneurysmal SAH. Recognition of pathophysiologic mechanisms of brain-body associations is essential in preventing complications after treatment of ruptured brain aneurysms.

The clinician should be vigilant about:

1. Maintenance of sodium and water balance,
2. Potential negative impact of agents which interfere with the renin-angiotensin-aldosterone system (including corticosteroids and angiotensin-converting enzyme inhibitors),
3. ventilatory support to overcome pulmonary edema, and
4. inotropic and vasopressor support for the stunned myocardium.

Pathophysiologic mechanisms for early-onset cerebral edema, as well as associations between brain-gastrointestinal and brain-immune systems will be elucidated in following sections.

References

[1] Audibert G, Steinmann G, de Talancé, et al. Endocrine responses after severe subarachnoid hemorrhage related to sodium and blood volume regulation. *Neurosurgical Anesthesiology and Neuroscience*. 2009 June; 108(6);1922-1928.

[2] Bederson JB. AANS Publications Committee. *Subarachnoid hemorrhage: pathophysiology and management.* Park Ridge, Ill.: American Association of Neurological Surgeons, 1997.

[3] Bewseoglu K, Holtkamp K, Steiger HJ, et al. Fatal aneurysmal subarachnoid hemorrhage. *Clinical Neurology and Neurosurgery.* 2013;115:77-81.

[4] Ebihara T, Kinoshita K, Utagawa A, et al. Changes in coagulative *and fibrinolytic activities in patients with intracranial hemorrhage. Acta Neurochir.* 2006 (Suppl);96:69-73.

[5] Espiner E, Leikis R, Ferch R, et al. The neuro-cardio-endocrine response to acute subarachnoid hemorrhage. *Clinical Endocrinology.* 2002; 56:629-635.

[6] Inamasu J, Nakatsukasa M, Mayanagi K, et al. Subarachnoid hemorrhage complicated with neurogenic pulmonary edema and Tako-tsubo-like cardiomyopathy. *Neurol Med Chir* (Tokyo). 2012; 52:49-55.

[7] Junttila E, Koskenkari J, Romppainen N, et al. Risk factors for 1-year mortality in patients with nontraumatic intracranial hemorrhage requiring intensive care. *Acta Anesthesiol Scand.* 2011;55:1052-1060.

[8] Kamath M, Watanabe M, *Upton ARM. Heart rate variability (HRV) signal analysis: clinical applications.* Boca Raton: Taylor & Francis, 2013.

[9] Kudo K, Konta T, Degawa N, et al. Relationship between kidney damage and stroke types in Japanese patients. *Clin Exp Nephrol.* 2012;16:564-569.

[10] Lo BWY, Fukuda H, Angle M, et al. Clinical outcome prediction in aneurysmal subarachnoid hemorrhage - Alterations in brain-body interface. *Surg Neurol Int.* 2016 Aug 1;7(Suppl 18):S527-37.

[11] Lo BWY, Fukuda H, Angle M, et al. Aneurysmal subarachnoid hemorrhage prognostic decision-making algorithm using classification and regression tree analysis. *Surg Neurol Int.* 2016 Jul 7;7:73.

[12] Lo BWY, Fukuda H, Nishimura Y, et al. *Brain-body interactions: contemporary outcome prediction in aneurysmal subarachnoid*

hemorrhage using bayesian neural networks and fuzzy logic. New York: Nova Biomedical, 2014.

[13] Lo BWY, Fukuda H, Nishimura Y, et al. Pathophysiologic mechanisms of brain-body associations in ruptured brain aneurysms: A systematic review. *Surg Neurol Int*. 2015 Aug 11;6:136.

[14] Naidech A, Kreiter K, Janjua N, et al. Cardiac troponin elevation, cardiovascular morbidity and outcome after subarachnoid hemorrhage. *Circulation*. 2005; 112:2851-2856.

[15] Nakamura T, Okuchi K, Matsuyama T, et al. Clinical significance of elevated natriuretic peptide levels and cardiopulmonary parameters after subarachnoid hemorrhage. *Neurol Med Chir* (Tokyo). 2009; 49:185-192.

[16] Sato Y, Isotani E, Kubota Y, et al. Circulatory characteristics of normovolemia and normotension therapy after subarachnoid hemorrhage, focusing on pulmonary edema. *Acta Neurochir*. 2012; 154:2195-2202.

[17] Whiting P, Rutjes A, Westwood M, et al. QUADAS-2: A revised tool for the quality assessment of diagnostic accuracy studies. *Annals of Internal Medicine* 2011;155:529-536.

[18] Zacharia B, Ducruet A, Hickman Z, et al. Renal dysfunction as an independent predictor of outcome after aneurysmal subarachnoid hemorrhage. *Stroke*. 2009;40:2375-2381.

[19] Zygun D, Doig C, Gupta A, et al. Non-neurological organ dysfunction in neurocritical care. *Journal of Critical Care*. 2003 December;18(4):238-244.

Section Two

Systematic Review of Prognostic Factors in Aneurysmal Subarachnoid Hemorrhage

Benjamin W. Y. Lo[1,*], Hitoshi Fukuda[2] and Mitchell A. H. Levine[3]

[1]Departments of Neurosurgery,
Neurology and Critical Care Medicine, Montreal Neurological Institute and Hospital, McGill University, Montreal, Canada
[2]Department of Neurosurgery,
Kochi University Hospital, Kochi, Japan
[3]Department of Clinical Epidemiology and Biostatistics (Department of Health Research Methods, Evidence and Impact), Department of Medicine, Division of Clinical Pharmacology, Centre for Evaluation of Medicines, St. Joseph's Hospital, McMaster University, Hamilton, Ontario, Canada

[*] Corresponding Author Email: benjamin.lo@mcgill.ca.

Introduction

Clinical prediction tools assist in clinical outcome prediction. This systematic review synthesizes and critically appraises methodologic quality of studies that derive both clinical predictors and clinical predictor tools used to determine outcome prognosis in patients suffering from aneurysmal SAH.

Clinical Prediction Tools

Clinical prediction tools assist in clinical outcome prediction, in establishing the likelihood of presence or absence of a condition, as well as in determining potential therapeutic courses of action. As such, they complement clinical opinion and judgment. Clinical prediction tools quantify the relative contributions of certain variables and condense information that identifies important indicators or predictors to a targeted condition [1-6, 12, 19, 31, 35, 36].

Methodologic assessment of clinical prediction tools pertains to their derivation and validation. In their development, the study from which the database is developed is critiqued for its study protocol (including inclusion and exclusion criteria, setting, patient recruitment, effective power with sample size for each predictor variable, description of patient characteristics and follow-up, report and handling of missing data, and subgroup analyses), relevance of predictor variables and outcomes studied (justification and definition of variables and outcomes used, with attention to their coding and reproducibility), and description of mathematical models (whether these models are both statistically and clinically sensible). In terms of model performance and validation, clinical prediction tools should be presented with a discussion of the types of performance measures used, as well as the types of validation used (including internal validation techniques such as data splitting, boot-strapping, and external validation techniques, like adopting the derived rules in an external population) [1-6, 12, 19, 31, 35, 36].

Aneurysmal Subarachnoid Hemorrhage

Intracranial aneurysmal subarachnoid hemorrhage (SAH) affects about 45,000 individuals in North America and 600,000 individuals worldwide annually. Aneurysmal SAH is associated with a morality rate of at least 45% in the first 30 days following rupture [22]. Apart from the primary neurological injury from the aneurysmal rupture itself, other secondary injury processes can further worsen an individual's neurological condition and eventual clinical outcome. These processes include both neurological processes (such as delayed stroke, re-bleeding, brain swelling, vasospasm induced strokes, seizures and hydrocephalus) and systemic medical complications (such as myocardial infarction, fever and pulmonary edema) [13, 21, 22]. Together, these processes can lead to long-term disability. Types of disability include physical, neurocognitive and psychological impairment. Long-term reductions in health-related quality of life are common, even though the case fatality of aneurysmal SAH has slowly declined due to prompt diagnosis and repair, as well as improved critical care medical management [13, 21, 22].

Objectives

The purpose of this systematic review is to synthesize and critically appraise methodologic quality of studies that derive both clinical predictor tools and clinical predictors used to determine outcome prognosis in patients suffering from aneurysmal SAH, with inclusion of studies with data generated from both prospective and retrospective cohort studies, and randomized controlled trials (RCTs).

Methods

This systematic review was designed based on a predefined protocol.

Study Eligibility Criteria

We included prospective and retrospective cohort studies, and RCTs investigating clinical prediction tools and prognostic factors associated with determining neurologic outcome in adult patients with aneurysmal SAH. We excluded prognostic studies and grading schemes based on expert opinions, those for traumatic SAH and perimesencephalic SAH. Eligible studies were limited to those published from January 1, 1995 to March 31, 2014, due to differences in diagnostic modalities and treatment prior to this point.

Literature Search

Two reviewers (Benjamin Lo [BL], Hitoshi Fukuda [HF]) independently searched a number of electronic databases. Relevant studies were identified from Ovid MEDLINE, Ovid EMBASE, Web of Science, the Cumulative Index to Nursing and Allied Health Literature, without language restrictions. To include gray literature, we also searched ProceedingsFirst and PapersFirst. We used the following search terms:

1. "aneurysmal subarachnoid hemorrhage" and "clinical prognosis,"
2. "aneurysmal subarachnoid hemorrhage" and "prediction rules."

Study Selection and Data Collection Process

Investigators (BL and HF) reviewed all titles and abstracts, and full reports of all potentially relevant trials. The initial literature search (January 1, 1995 to March 31, 2014) yielded 2863 citations (Figure 2.1). Screening by title and abstract yielded 121 items. Of these 121 items, reviewers BL and HF reached agreement on 70 items for inclusion (prospective and retrospective cohort studies, and RCTs investigating clinical prediction tools and prognostic factors associated with determining neurologic outcome in adult patients with aneurysmal SAH), 42 items for exclusion (prognostic studies and grading schemes based on expert opinions, studies for traumatic SAH and perimesencephalic SAH), and were unsure on 9 items. Inter-rater reliability was high (estimated kappa 0.85 (95% confidence interval [CI] 0.80-0.90) for citation and abstract screening).

Seventy-nine full-text articles were identified as potentially relevant and were assessed with further exclusion of articles due to incomplete variable and outcome reporting (n = 13), inappropriate patient inclusion and exclusion criteria (n = 18), and inappropriate predictor models used (n = 26) [Figure 2.1].

Investigators BL and HF then independently applied the inclusion criteria to the full reports. Each trial report was examined carefully for its methodologic quality. As outlined in the "methodologic quality assessment" section, each article was appraised in nine areas. Of the 198 items assessed in 22 articles, BL and HF reached agreement on 160 items, disagreed on 30 items and were unsure on 8 items (kappa statistic 0.85, 95% CI 0.80-0.90).

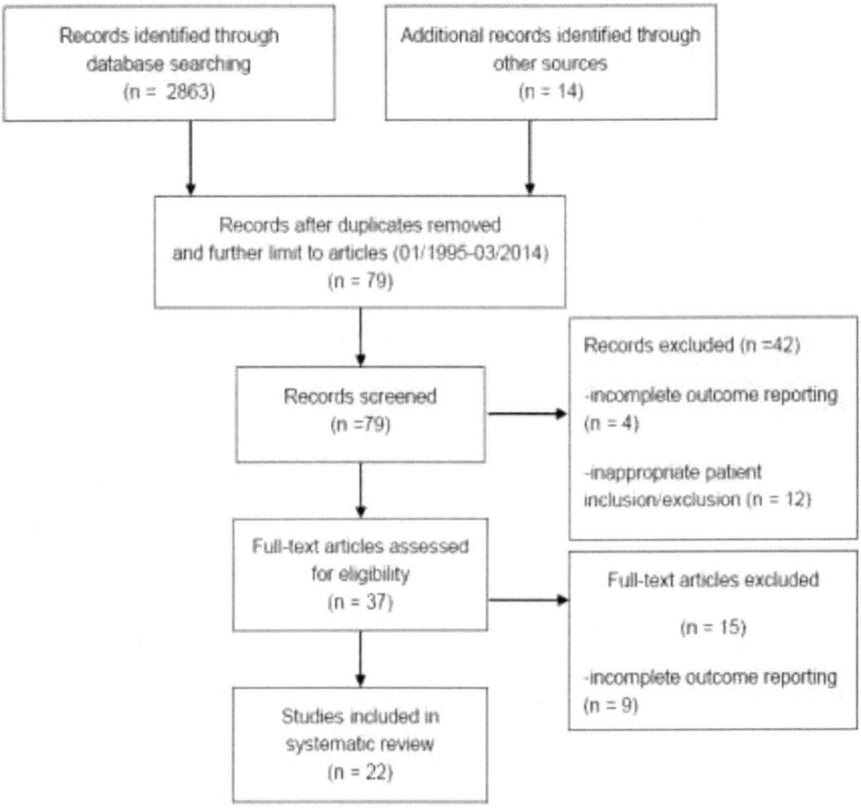

Figure 2.1. Flow diagram of study selection.

Methodologic Quality Assessment

For this systematic review, we sampled the quality checklist using Delphi methods for clinical prediction rules (QUADCPR) [9], and criteria proposed by Bouwmeester et al. 2012 [5] for methodologic quality assessment of clinical prediction research. The following areas were used in methodologic quality assessment:

1. study design – including description of study protocol, inclusion and exclusion criteria, study setting and recruitment,

2. patient population – including representativeness of exposed aneurysmal subarachnoid hemorrhage patient cohort and ascertainment of exposure,
3. candidate predictors – including description of predictors (neurologic, systemic and demographic variables) used, selection and coding of data, inclusion of potential confounding variables,
4. outcome – including definition of outcomes (neurological and functional outcomes), justification of outcomes, their reproducibility, length of follow-up and outcome assessment when appropriate,
5. statistical power – ensuring effective sample size,
6. statistical models – description of mathematical methods used, and whether they are statistically sound and clinically sensible,
7. bias assessment – such as publication bias, selection bias, recall bias, referral bias, and ascertainment bias,
8. model performance and validation – descriptions of any attempts to evaluate, if appropriate, model performance and validation, and
9. statement of conflict of interest or funding.

Results

Study Search and Selection

The initial literature search (January 1, 1995 – March 31, 2014) yielded 2863 citations (Figure 2.1). These were screened by title and abstract. Seventy-nine full-text articles were identified as potentially relevant and were assessed with the further exclusion of articles due to an incomplete variable and outcome reporting, inappropriate patient inclusion and exclusion criteria, an inappropriate predictor models used.

Twenty-two studies were included in this systemic review, with Table 2.1 examining the independent, confounding and outcome variables, and Table 2.2 examining their methodologic quality.

Study Results and Synthesis of Results

This systemic review of both clinical prediction tools and prognostic factors in patients with aneurysmal SAH comprised 3 studies analyzing databases from RCTs, 8 prospective cohort studies, and 11 retrospective cohort studies. The most frequently retained significant clinical prognostic factors for long-term neurologic outcome prediction include age (n = 7: Germanson et al. 1998 [10], McGirt et al. 2007 [23], Ogilvy et al. 2006 [28], Rabinstein et al. 2004 [30], Risselada et al. 2010 [32], Rosengart et al. 2007[33], Karamanakos et al. 2012 [16]), neurological grade (n = 6: Germanson et al. 1998 [10], Kahn et al. 2006 [15], McGirt et al. 2007 [23], Ogilvy et al. 2006 [28], Rabinstein et al. 2004 [30], Risselada et al. 2010 [32], Karamanakos et al. 2012 [16]), blood clot thickness on CT imaging (n = 4: Ogilvy et al. 2006 [28], Rabinstein et al. 2004 [30], Risselada et al. 2010 [32], Rosengart et al. 2007 [33]), and aneurysm size (n = 2: Rosengart et al. 2007 [33], Risselada et al. 2010 [32]). Table 2.1 describes the aforementioned variables depicted in individual studies.

Methodological Quality of Included Studies

The included 22 studies all had thorough descriptions of study protocols, including inclusion and exclusion criteria. Representative patient cohorts were included in these studies. 4 of the 22 studies included multicenter cohorts. With the exception of one study (Soehle et al. 2007 [34]), all studies had adequate patient sample sizes to ensure effective study power, ensuring 10 outcome events per variable investigated. Predictor variables were adequately defined in all studies. Patients were followed from 1 to 12 months after aneurysmal rupture for assessment of neurological outcomes, with small proportions of patients lost to follow-up. Neurologic and functional outcome assessments were performed in 15 of 22 studies. In addition, most studies (19 of 22 studies) accounted for potential confounding variables and stratification in their analyses (Tables 2.1 and 2.2). Univariate and multivariable logistic regression analyses were used for most studies (21 of 22 studies). However, only 6 of 22 studies checked for model performance including good calibration (agreement between predicted probabilities and observed outcome frequencies) and good discrimination (ability to distinguish between patients with and without the outcome) [2-4]. Finally, studies of clinical predictors and prediction models in aneurysmal SAH are prone to patient selection and referral biases, as well as recall bias in outcome assessments (Table 2.2).

Discussion

This systematic review was conducted to synthesize current evidence on prognostic factors affecting the outcome in aneurysmal SAH and to appraise the methodologic quality of studies investigating these clinical outcome prediction tools.

Methodological Issues

Systematic reviews for clinical prognostic factors and clinical prediction tools in aneurysmal SAH face a number of methodological challenges. These include within and between study patient heterogeneity, regional variations in treatment protocols, patient referral biases, and differences in treatment and prognosis viewpoints across different cultures.

Between-center differences in treatment and patient populations influence patient prognosis and clinical outcomes [7, 8, 10, 11, 14-18, 20, 22-30, 32-34, 37, 38]. These center cluster effects should be taken into account when determining the effect sizes of individual prognostic factors. In addition, prognostic variables may be co-dependent [7, 8, 10, 11, 14-18, 20, 22-30, 32-34, 37, 38]. Exploration of interactions between variables is important as they reflect the interrelated pathophysiologic mechanisms of brain-body associations in aneurysmal SAH.

Unlike a recently performed systematic review on clinical prediction models in aneurysmal SAH [13], this systematic review included:

1. studies that provide clear definitions of predictor variables,
2. studies with adequate study effective power and sample sizes, and
3. methodological assessment based on standardized guidelines for quality assessment of clinical prediction tools.

This systematic review also attempted to overcome other methodological limitations by including high quality cohort studies and RCTs in prognosis fulfilling a number of quality assessment criteria, namely, those proposed by QUADCPR [9], and criteria proposed by Bouwmeester et al. 2012 [5]. In addition, all included studies had clearly defined predictor and outcome variables, effective study power, as well as clinically and statistically sensible prediction tools and prognostic factors. Across most studies, the core and most frequently retained clinical outcome predictors in aneurysmal SAH include age [10, 16, 23, 8, 30, 32, 33], neurological grade [10, 15, 16, 23, 28, 30, 32], aneurysm size [32, 33] and blood clot thickness [28, 30, 32, 33].

Table 2.1. Variables investigated in existing clinical prognostic models in aneurysmal subarachnoid hemorrhage

	Independent Variables	**Independent Variables Controlled for during Analysis**	**Dependent Variables**
Chiang et al. [7]	-worst clinical grade (WFNS, Hunt and Hess) before treatment	-age	-outcome (Glasgow Outcome Scale, Karnofsky scale)
Claassen et al. [8]	-hypoxia (arterio-alveolar gradient > 125 mmHg) -metabolic acidosis (bicarbonate < 20 mmol/L) -hyperglycemia (glucose > 180 mg/dL) -cardiovascular instability (mean arterial pressure < 70 or > 130 mmHg)	-in hospital rebleeding -aneurysm size -intraventricular hemorrhage -level of consciousness at onset -age	-poor outcome (modified Rankin Score > 3)
Germanson et al. [10]	-age -sex -preexisting hypertension -aneurysm size and location -CT clot thickness -serum glucose -Glasgow Coma Score -level of consciousness	-none	-outcome (Glasgow Outcome Score at 3 months)

Table 2.1. (Continued)

	Independent Variables	Independent Variables Controlled for during Analysis	Dependent Variables
Heuer et al. [11]	-neurological grade (Hunt and Hess grade, GCS motor score) -intracerebral hemorrhage -intraventricular hemorrhage -rebleeding -intraoperative cerebral swelling -postoperative GCS score	-age -aneurysm size -vasospasm -intraoperative aneurysm rupture -secondary cerebral insults	-increased intracranial pressure -lack of correlation between intracranial pressure and poor neurological outcome (Hunt and Hess grades 4 and 5)
Juvela [14]	-clinical condition at admission (GCS) -rebleeding -delayed cerebral ischemia -surgical clipping -heavy consumption of alcohol	-sex -age	-poor outcome (Glasgow Outcome Score 1-3)
Kahn et al. [15]	-severity of illness -clinical grade of hemorrhage -red blood cell transfusions -severe sepsis	-intracranial pressure -cerebral perfusion pressure -Hunt and Hess grade	-acute lung injury -mortality
Kramer et al. [17]	-late pulmonary infiltrates (> 72 hours) -early pulmonary infiltrates (< 72 hours)	-age -initial WFNS grade -amount of blood on initial CT -presence of symptomatic vasospasm	-poor outcome (Glasgow Outcome Score 1-3) -mortality

	Independent Variables	**Independent Variables Controlled for during Analysis**	**Dependent Variables**
Krishnamurthy et al. [18]	-smoking	-age -sex -Hunt and Hess grade -amount of blood on initial CT (Fisher grade) -medical comorbidities	-poor outcome (Glasgow Outcome Score 1-3) -delayed neurological deterioration
Lindvall et al. [20]	-amount of blood of CT (Fisher grade) -Hunt and Hess grade	-age	-poor outcome (Glasgow Outcome Score 1-3)
McGirt e al. [23]	-glucose level	-Hunt and Hess grade -cerebral vasospasm -age -hypertension -ventriculomegaly on CT	-poor outcome (Glasgow Outcome Score 1 to 3)
Miss et al. [24]	-aneurysm coiling -aneurysm clipping	-hemodynamic factors -mechanical ventilation -phenylephrine doses	-cardiac troponin I > 1.0 mcg/L -regional wall motion abnormalities -left ventricular ejection fraction < 50%

Table 2.1. (Continued)

	Independent Variables	Independent Variables Controlled for during Analysis	Dependent Variables
Mocco et al. [25]	-age -hyperglycemia -worst preoperative Hunt and Hess grades (4 and 5) -aneurysm size (> 13 mm)	-sex -medical history (obesity, hypertension, myocardial infarction, coronary artery disease, congestive heart failure, arrhythmia, diabetes, renal disease, stroke, depression, anxiety disorder, smoking) -hemoglobin level -leukocytosis -sodium level -acute pulmonary disease -aneurysm coiling -aneurysm clipping -acute hydrocephalus -global cerebral edema -intracerebral hemorrhage	-poor neurologic outcome (Hunt and Hess grade 5, mortality)
Naidech et al. [26]	-hemoglobin level	-Hunt and Hess grade -age -angiographic vasospasm	-cerebral infarction -poor outcome (Hunt and Hess grades 4 and 5)

	Independent Variables	**Independent Variables Controlled for during Analysis**	**Dependent Variables**
Ogilvy et al. [28]	-Hunt and Hess grade -Fisher grade -aneurysm size -age -anterior circulation aneurysms	-aneurysm clipping -aneurysm coiling -posterior circulation aneurysms	-poor outcome (Hunt and Hess grades 4 and 5)
Qureshi et al. [29]	-sodium level	-age, sex -pre-existing hypertension -admission neurological grade (GCS score) -initial mean arterial pressure -subarachnoid clot thickness -intraventricular blood -intraparenchymal hematoma -ventricular dilation -aneurysm size and location	-outcome (Glasgow Outcome Scale, mortality rate)
Rabinstein et al. [30]	-age -initial WFNS grade -coiling	-anterior aneurysm location -global deficits -diffuse vasospasm -number of affected vessels -number of endovascular treatments	-poor outcome (WFNS grades 4 and 5)
Risselada et al. [32]	-age -sex -prior subarachnoid hemorrhage	-randomization group	-outcome (Modified Rankin Scale, death at 2 months)

Table 2.1. (Continued)

	Independent Variables	Independent Variables Controlled for during Analysis	Dependent Variables
Risselada et al. [32]	-Fisher grade -lumbar puncture finding -WFNS grade -number of aneurysms -size and aneurysm location -vasospasm on admission	-randomization group	-outcome (Modified Rankin Scale, death at 2 months)
Rosengart et al. [33]	-age -admission neurological grade -clot thickness -aneurysm location -aneurysm size -systolic blood pressure -prior SAH -history of hypertension -intraventricular hemorrhage -anticonvulsant use -induced hypertension, hypervolemia hypervolemia -symptomatic vasospasm -fever at day 8 -cerebral infarction		-outcome (Glasgow Outcome Scale)

	Independent Variables	Independent Variables Controlled for during Analysis	Dependent Variables
Soehle et al. [34]	-poor initial neurologic grade (Hunt and Hess grade 4 or 5) -amount of blood on CT (Fisher grade) -pulsatility index -resistance index	-mean arterial blood pressure -intracranial pressure -middle cerebral artery flow velocity	-poor outcome (Glasgow Outcome Score 1 to 3)
Van den Bergh et al. [37]	-magnesium level -amounts of cisternal and ventricular blood	-duration of unconsciousness -sex -rebleeding -level of consciousness at admission	-poor outcome (WFNS grades 4 and 5)
Yoshimoto et al. [38]	-systemic inflammation (> 2 criteria)	-age -aneurysm location -amount of blood on CT (Fisher grade) -age -Hunt and Hess grade -glucose concentration	-poor outcome (Glasgow Outcome Score grades 1, 2 and 3)
Karamanakos et al. [16]	-age -Hunt and Hess grade -hydrocephalus	-gender -family history of saccular aneurysms -time period of aneurysmal SAH -intracerebral hemorrhage -intraventricular hemorrhage -subdural hematoma	-mortality at 1-3 days, mortality at 4-30 days, mortality at 1-12 months period

Table 2.2. Methodological assessment of clinical prognostic models on aneurysmal subarachnoid hemorrhage

Study Design	Chiang et al.	Claassen et al.	Germanson	Heuer et al.	Juvela	Kahn et al.
	Retrospective cohort	Retrospective cohort	Analysis of RCT database	Retrospective cohort	Prospective cohort	Retrospective cohort
Representativeness of cohort	Yes	Yes	Yes	Yes	Yes	Yes
Confounding	No adjustment	Adjusted	No adjustment	Adjusted	Adjusted	Adjusted
Blinding of assessors	No	Yes	Yes	Yes	No	Yes
Stratification	No	Yes	Yes	Yes	Yes	Yes
Statistical Methods & Sample Size	Univariate > 10 subjects per variable	Univariate Multivariable > 10 subjects per variable	Univariate Multivariable CART > 10 subjects per variable	Univariate Multivariable > 10 subjects per variable	Univariate Multivariable > 10 subjects per variable	Univariate Multivariable > 10 subjects per variable
Model Performance	None	C-statistic	None	None	Hosmer-Lemeshow	Hosmer-Lemeshow
Bias	Recall bias	No major	No major	Ascertainment bias	Recall bias	No major
Conflict of Interest Statement	Not stated	Declared	Declared	Not stated	Declared	Declared

Study Design	Kramer et al.	Krishnamurthy	Lindvall et al.	McGirt et al.	Miss et al.	Mocco et al.
	Retrospective cohort	Retrospective cohort	Prospective cohort	Retrospective cohort	Prospective cohort	Prospective cohort
Representativeness of cohort	Yes	Yes	Yes	Yes	Yes	Yes
Confounding	Adjusted	Adjusted	No adjustment	Adjusted	Adjusted	Adjusted
Blinding of assessors	Yes	No	Yes	Yes	Yes	Yes
Stratification	Yes	Yes	No	Yes	Yes	Yes
Statistical Methods & Sample Size	Univariate Multivariable 10 subjects per variable	Univariate Multivariable > 10 subjects per variable	Univariate Multivariable > 10 subjects per variable	Univariate Multivariable > 10 subjects per variable	Univariate Multivariable > 10 subjects per variable	Univariate Multivariable > 10 subjects per variable
Model Performance	None	None	C-statistic	None	None	None
Bias	No major	Recall bias Selection bias	No major	No major	No major	Selection bias Referral bias
Conflict of Interest Statement	Declared	Not stated	Declared	Declared	Declared	Declared

Table 2.2. (Continued)

Study Design	Naidech et al.	Ogilvy et al.	Qureshi et al.	Rabinstein et al.	Risselada et al.	Rosengart et al.
	Retrospective cohort	Prospective cohort	Retrospective cohort	Retrospective cohort	Analysis of RCT database	Analysis of RCT database
Representativeness of cohort	Yes	Yes	Yes	Yes	Yes	Yes
Confounding	Adjusted	Adjusted	Adjusted	Adjusted	Adjusted	Adjusted
Blinding of assessors	Yes	Yes	Yes	Yes	Yes	Yes
Stratification	Yes	Yes	Yes	Yes	Yes	Yes
Statistical Methods & Sample Size	Univariate Multivariable >10 subjects per variable	Univariate Multivariable >10 subjects per variable	Univariate Multivariable >10 subjects per variable	Univariate Multivariable 10 subjects per variable	Univariate Multivariable >10 subjects per variable	Univariate Multivariable >10 subjects per variable
Validation	None	None	None	None	Bootstrap Hosmer-Lemeshow C-statistic	Goodness of fit - McFadden R squared
Bias	No major	No major	No major	No major	No major	No major
Funding	Declared	Not stated	Not stated	Not stated	Declared	Declared

Study Design	Soehle et al.	van den Bergh et al.	Yoshimoto et al.	Karamanakos et al.
	Prospective cohort	Prospective cohort	Retrospective cohort	Prospective cohort
Representativeness of cohort	Yes	Yes	Yes	Yes
Confounding	Adjusted	Adjusted	Adjusted	Adjusted
Blinding of assessors	No	Not stated	Not stated	No
Stratification	No	Yes	Yes	Yes
Statistical Methods & Sample Size	Univariate Multivariable <10 subjects per variable	Univariate Multivariable >10 subjects per variable	Univariate Multivariable >10 subjects per variable	Univariate Multivariable >10 subjects per variable
Validation	None	None	None	None
Bias	No major	No major	Selection bias Referral bias	No major
Funding	Declared	Not stated	Not stated	Declared

Yet, a number of other systemic, physiologic and neurologic parameters may also turn out to be important clinical outcome predictors. These factors are usually not as frequently included in clinical outcome prognostic studies on aneurysmal SAH. For instance, even though the majority of studies (n = 20) used univariate and multivariable logistic regression analyses for determination of significant prognostic factors and clinical prediction tools, only 6 of 22 studies checked for model performance. In addition, model performance may be affected by interactions between core predictors, as well as latent variables not accounted for during analysis.

Conclusion

Studies attempting to elucidate prognostic factors in aneurysmal SAH are affected by a number of methodologic limitations. This systematic review attempted to overcome some of these methodologic limitations by synthesizing high-quality RCTs and cohort studies. Yet, these synthesized epidemiologic studies did not attempt to clarify underlying mechanisms of how ruptured brain aneurysms influence other body systems. Brain-body associations carry a significant impact on patients' clinical outcomes. Together, existing methodologic limitations of epidemiologic studies on outcome prognosis in aneurysmal SAH readily influence the quality of clinical insight gained in this area.

References

[1] Adams S, Leveson S. Clinical prediction rules. *BMJ.* 2012 Jan 16;344.

[2] Altman D, Royston P. What do we mean by validating a prognostic model? *Stat Med.* 2000 Feb 29; 19(4):453-473.

[3] Bartfay E, Bartfay W. Accuracy assessment of prediction in patient outcomes. *J Eval Clin Pract.* 2008 Feb; 14(1):1-10.

[4] Beattie P, Nelson R. Clinical prediction rules: what are they and what do they tell us? *Aust J Physiother.* 2006; 52(3):157-63.

[5] Bouwmeester W, Zuithoff N, Mallett S, et al. Reporting and methods in clinical prediction research: a systematic review. *PLoS Med.* 2012; 9(5):1-12.

[6] Brismee J, Sizer P. Potential pitfalls of clinical prediction rules. *J Man Manip Ther.* 2008;16(3):182.

[7] Chiang V, Claus E, Awad I. Toward more rational prediction of outcome in patients with high-grade subarachnoid hemorrhage. *Neurosurgery.* 2000;46(1):28-36.

[8] Claassen J, Vu A, Kreiter K, et al. Effect of acute physiologic derangements on outcome after subarachnoid hemorrhage. *Critical Care Med.* 2004;32(3):832-838.

[9] Cook C, Brismee J, Pietrobon R, et al. Development of a quality checklist using delphi methods for prescriptive clinical prediction rules: the QUADCPR. *J Manipulative Physiol Ther.* 2010 Jan;33(1):29-41.

[10] Germanson T, Lanzino G, Kongable G, et al. Risk classification after aneurysmal subarachnoid hemorrhage. *Surg Neurol.* 1998 Feb;49(2): 155-63.

[11] Heuer G, Smith M, Elliott J, et al. Relationship between intracranial pressure and other clinical variables in patients with aneurysmal subarachnoid hemorrhage. *J Neurosurg.* 2004;101:408-416.

[12] Hier D, Edelstein G. Deriving clinical prediction rules from stroke outcome research. *Stroke.* 1991 Nov; 22(11):1431-6.

[13] Jaja BN, Cusimano M, Etminan N, et al. Clinical prediction models for aneurysmal subarachnoid hemorrhage: a systematic review. *Neurocritic Care* 2013;18(1),143-153.

[14] Juvela S. Alcohol consumption as a risk factor for poor outcome after aneurysmal subarachnoid haemorrhage. *BMJ.* 1992; 304:1663-1667.

[15] Kahn J, Caldwell E, Deem S, et al. Acute lung injury in patients with subarachnoid hemorrhage: incidence, risk factors and outcome. *Crit Care Med.* 2006;34(1):196-202.

[16] Karamankos P, von Und Zu Fraunberg M, Bendel S, et al. Risk factors for three phases of 12-month mortality in 1657 patients from a defined population after acute aneurysmal subarachnoid hemorrhage. *World Neurosurg* 2012;78:631-9.

[17] Kramer A, Bleck T, Dumont A, et al. Implications of early versus late bilateral pulmonary infiltrates in patients with aneurysmal subarachnoid hemorrhage. *Neurocritical Care.* 2009;10:20-27.

[18] Krishnamurthy S, Kelleher J, Lehman E, et al. Effects of tobacco dose and length of exposure on delayed neurological deterioration and overall clinical outcome after aneurysmal subarachnoid hemorrhage. *Neurosurgery.* 2007;61(3):475-481.

[19] Laupacis A, Sekar N, Stiell I. Clinical prediction rules. A review and suggested modifications of methodological standards. *JAMA.* 1997 Feb 12;277(6):488-94.

[20] Lindvall P, Runnerstam M, Birgander R, et al. The Fisher grading correlated to outcome in patients with subarachnoid hemorrhage. *British Journal of Neurosurgery.* 2009;23(2):188-192.

[21] Lo B, Macdonald RL. Health related quality of life after aneurysmal subarachnoid hemorrhage: new data from a large series in Germany. *World Neurosurg.* 2013 Feb;79(2):243-4.

[22] Macdonald R, Cusimano M, Etminan N, et al. Subarachnoid hemorrhage international trialists data repository (SAHIT). *World Neurosurg.* 2013 Mar-Apr;79(3-4):481-22.

[23] McGirt M, Woodworth G, Ali M, et al. Persistent perioperative hyperglycemia as an independent predictor of poor outcome after aneurysmal subarachnoid hemorrhage. *J Neurosurg.* 2007; 107:1080-1085.
[24] Miss J, Kopelnik A, Fisher L, et al. Cardiac injury after subarachnoid hemorrhage is independent of the type of aneurysm therapy. *Neurosurgery.* 2004;55(6):1244-1251.
[25] Mocco J, Ransom E, Komotar R, et al. Preoperative prediction of long-term outcome in poor-grade aneurysmal subarachnoid hemorrhage. *Neurosurgery.* 2006;59(3):529-538.
[26] Naidech A, Drescher J, Ault M, et al. Higher hemoglobin is associated with less cerebral infarction, poor outcome, and death after subarachnoid hemorrhage. *Neurosurgery.* 2006;59(4):775-779.
[27] Naidech A, Janjua N, Kreiter K, et al. Predictors and impact of aneurysm rebleeding after subarachnoid hemorrhage. *Arch Neurol.* 2005;62:410-416.
[28] Ogilvy C, Cheung A, Mitha A, et al. Outcomes for surgical and endovascular management of intracranial aneurysms using a comprehensive grading system. *Neurosurgery.* 2006;59(5):1037-1042.
[29] Qureshi A, Suri F, Sung G, et al. Prognostic significance of hypernatremia and hyponatremia among patients with aneurysmal subarachnoid hemorrhage. *Neurosurgery.* 2002;50(4):749-755.
[30] Rabinstein A, Friedman J, Nichols D, et al. Predictors of outcome after endovascular treatment of cerebral vasospasm. *Am J Neuroradiol.* 2004;25:1778-1782.
[31] Raymond J, Naggara O, Guilbert F, et al. Assessing prognosis from nonrandomized studies: an example from brain arteriovenous malformations. *AJNR Am J Neuroradiol.* 2011 May;32(5):809-12.

[32] Risselada R, Lingsma H, Bauer-MehrenA, et al. Prediction of 60 day case-fatality after aneurysmal subarachnoid haemorrhage: results from the International Subarachnoid Aneurysm Trial (ISAT). *Eur J Epidemiol.* 2010 April;25(4):261-6.

[33] Rosengart A, Schultheiss K, Tolentino J, et al. Prognostic factors for outcome in patients with aneurysmal subarachnoid hemorrhage. *Stroke.* 2007; 38(8):2315-21.

[34] Soehle M, Chatfield D, Czosnyka M, et al. Predictive value of initial clinical status, intracranial pressure and transcranial doppler pulsatility after subarachnoid hemorrhage. *Acta Neurochir (Wien)* 2007;149:575-583.

[35] Steyerberg E, Vickers A, Cook N, et al. Assessing the performance of prediction models: a framework for traditional and novel measures. *Epidemiology.* 2010 Jan;21(1):128-38.

[36] Toll D, Janssen K, Vergouwe Y, et al. Validation, updating and impact of clinical prediction rules: a review. *J Clin Epidemiol.* 2008 Nov;61(11):1085-94.

[37] van den Bergh W, Algra A, van der Sprenkel J, et al. Hypomagnesemia after aneurysmal subarachnoid hemorrhage. *Neurosurgery.* 2003;52(2):276-282.

[38] Yoshimoto Y, Tanaka Y, Hoya K. Acute systemic inflammatory response syndrome in subarachnoid hemorrhage. *Stroke.* 2001;32:1989-1993.

Section Three

Alterations in Brain-Body Interface in Aneurysmal Subarachnoid Hemorrhage – Comparative Regression Analyses in Two Cohorts

Benjamin W. Y. Lo[1,*], Hitoshi Fukuda[2], Masaomi Koyanagi[3], Adrian Upton[4] and Mitchell A. H. Levine[5]

[1]Departments of Neurosurgery,
Neurology and Critical Care Medicine,
Montreal Neurological Institute and Hospital,
McGill University, Montreal, Canada

[*] Corresponding Author Email: benjamin.lo@mcgill.ca.

[2]Department of Neurosurgery, Kochi University Hospital, Kochi, Japan
[3]Department of Neurosurgery, National Hospital Organization Himeji Medical Center, Himeji, Japan
[4]Division of Neurology, Department of Medicine, McMaster University, Hamilton, Ontario, Canada
[5]Department of Clinical Epidemiology and Biostatistics (Department of Health Research Methods, Evidence and Impact), Department of Medicine, Division of Clinical Pharmacology, Centre for Evaluation of Medicines, St. Joseph's Hospital, McMaster University, Hamilton, Ontario, Canada

Introduction

Brain-body associations are essential in influencing outcome in patients with ruptured brain aneurysms. The goal of this section is to use binary logistic regression to investigate potential factors for outcome prediction in patients with ruptured brain aneurysms, as well as interactions of these factors for possible associations between the brain and other organ systems. In so doing, novel insights will be shed on brain-body interactions in aneurysmal subarachnoid hemorrhage, as pathophysiologic correlations will be made.

Two patient cohorts will be used, namely, the multicenter Tirilazad database (3551 patients) and a contemporary database from Kurashiki Central Hospital, a stroke center affiliated with Kyoto University, Japan (504 patients).

Table 3.1 The brain-body interface under normal homeostasis and after aneurysmal subarachnoid hemorrhage

Cardiovascular System Under Normal Homeostasis -autonomic nervous control of cardiovascular system: 1. counter-regulatory feedback with sympathetic nervous system, and 2. primary relay station being vasomotor regions of the lower brainstem
Cardiovascular System Dysfunction in Aneurysmal SAH -altered autonomic nervous control of cardiovascular system: 1. sympathetic nervous system activation, 2. blood pressure changes sensed by carotid sinus baroreceptors, and 3. blood around lower brainstem triggers catecholamine release from thoracic paravertebral chain
Pulmonary System under Normal Homeostasis -automatic control of respiration by lower brainstem's pacemaker cells with additional modifications by: 1. brainstem chemoreceptors and vascular baroreceptors, 2. brain (limbic, hypothalamic and brainstem) inputs and spinal (cervical and thoracic cord) reflexes, and 3. pulmonary local volume and vascular controls
Pulmonary System Dysfunction in Aneurysmal SAH -altered autonomic control of respiration with sympathetic surge: 1. blood oxygen, carbon dioxide and pH levels change and sensed by chemoreceptors and baroreceptors, 2. altered brain and spinal inputs trigger hyperventilation and ataxic breathing patterns, and 3. increased pulmonary vascular permeability and venous pressures leading to hydrostatic pulmonary edema.
Endocrine System in Normal Homeostasis -hypothalamic-pituitary axis coordinates key aspects of homeostasis 1. counter-regulatory feedback with target end organs including the adrenal glands
Endocrinological System Dysfunction in Aneurysmal SAH -altered hypothalamic-pituitary axis: 1. sodium and water imbalance triggered by early altered levels of natriuretic peptides and later compensation by the renin-angiotensin-aldosterone system

The Tirilazad Database

Tirilazad was a 21-aminosteroid compound produced by Pharmacia and Upjohn, Kalamazoo, Michigan. It was originally investigated as a free radical scavenger for the potential treatment of cerebral vasospasm. Between 1991 and 1997, 3551 patients from 171 centers in 22 countries in North America, Europe, Australia, New Zealand and Africa participated in five randomized, double-blind, placebo-controlled trials of Tirilazad.

Included patients were adults with evidence of aneurysmal SAH. The patients received either placebo or active agent (in intravenous doses of 0.6, 2.6 or 15 mg/kg/day depending on the trial) from the third to tenth day after onset of SAH. Excluded patients were:

1. those with traumatic SAH,
2. those with infectious mycotic aneurysms,
3. severe underlying medical illnesses including serious cardiovascular disease, such as myocardial infarction within the previous 6 months, uncontrolled hypertension, serious cardiac arrthymias or congestive heart failure,
4. pregnant or lactating patients,
5. patients taking corticosteroids or calcium channel blockers other than nimodipine,
6. known intolerance to calcium channel blockers, and
7. patients whose aneurysms were treated with Guglielmi or other detachable coils.

Patients in the placebo and treatment arms were otherwise treated similarly. Over 85% of patients underwent surgical clipping, and half of them were operated within the first 48 hours. Baseline demographics in both arms were balanced in terms of sex, age, number of pre-existing medical conditions, mean time to treatment, mean admission systolic blood pressure, admission neurological grade, ruptured aneurysm location, amount of blood visualized on admission CT scan (measured by the Fisher scale taking into account thickness of blood clot with or without intraventricular component). The potential confounder of patient sex was accounted for in statistical analysis in the North American Tirilazad trial where fewer female patients were randomized to the treatment arm. The percentages of patients experiencing neurological and systemic disabilities were similar in different treatment groups.

Only one percent of patients were lost to follow up. The primary outcome measure was the patient's Glasgow Outcome Score at 3 months after aneurysmal rupture. Glasgow Outcome Score is a 5-point scale, defined as: 5 – good recovery with normal life activities despite minor deficits, 4 – moderate disability being disabled but independent, 3 – severe disability being conscious but dependent, 2 – persistent vegetative state, and 1 – death.

Among the five Tirilazad trials, no substantial heterogeneity was found, and no significant differences between treatment and placebo arms, or amongst patients who were administered different dosages of Tirilazad regarding the number of patients who died, the number of adverse events or neurological outcome at 3 months follow up.

The Kurashiki Central Hospital Aneurysmal Subarachnoid Hemorrhage Database

The Kurashiki Central Hospital aneurysmal subarachnoid hemorrhage database identified 504 patients with ruptured brain aneurysms from 2008-2015. This aSAH database captured four significant advances in the contemporary diagnosis and management of patients with ruptured brain aneusysms. They include:

1. early surgery for ruptured aneurysms based on diagnostic CT angiograms,
2. advanced contemporary surgical and endovascular techniques, including aneurysm clipping (Figure 3.1), aneurysm trapping with bypass (Figure 3.2), aneurysm coiling (Figure 3.3) and parent artery occlusion,
3. external decompression for a SAH patients with cerebral edema, and
4. advanced neurocritical care management to prevent and reduce the incidence of symptomatic vasospasm, including intravenous vasodilatory fasudil and brain cisternal flush using a combination of milrinone (vasodilatory drug), urokinase (for blood clot lysis) and ascorbic acid (water-soluble, antioxidant vitamin C).

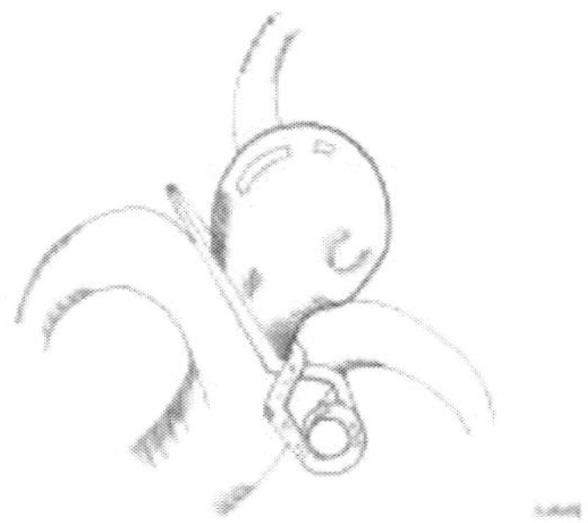

Figure 3.1. Cerebral aneurysm clipping.

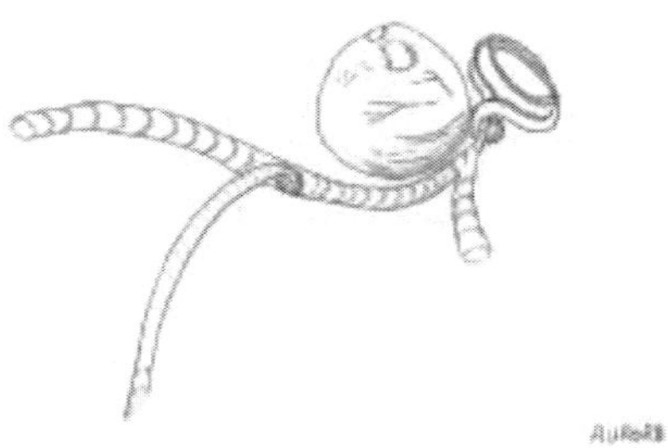

Figure 3.2. Cerebral aneurysm trapping and bypass.

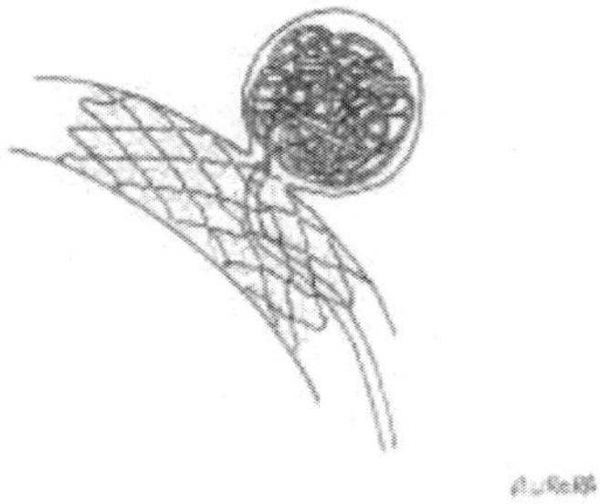

Figure 3.3. Cerebral aneurysm coiling.

Methods

The Tirilazad and Kurashiki Central Hospital databases were used to investigate the potential factors for outcome prediction in aneurysmal SAH and to assess interactions of factors between the brain and other organ systems.

Independent variables recorded in the Tirilizad database are listed as follows:

Demographic Risk Factors

1. age (in years),
2. sex,
3. patient's weight (kg)

Systemic Risk Factors

1. systolic blood pressure (mmHg),
2. diastolic blood pressure (mmHg),
3. temperature on admission (degree Celsius),

4. occurrence of fever one week after hospital admission,
5. history of hypertension,
6. history of angina,
7. history of myocardial infarction,
8. history of diabetes mellitus,
9. history of hepatic disease,
10. history of thyroid disease,
11. development of pulmonary edema

Non-Treatment Related Neurologic Risk Factors

1. hospital admission neurological grade (Hunt and Hess) [1 – asymptomatic, 2 – headaches, cranial nerve palsy, 3 – mild focal deficit, confusion, 4 – stupor, moderate to severe hemiparesis, 5 – deep coma, moribund],
2. aneurysm size (≤ 12 mm or > 12 mm),
3. presence of angiographic vasospasm on hospital admission,
4. presence of intraventricular hemorrhage,
5. presence of intracerebral hemorrhage,
6. location of aneurysm (anterior or posterior circulation),
7. thickness of subarachnoid hemorrhage (≤ 1 mm or > 1 mm),
8. prior episode of subarachnoid hemorrhage,
9. history of migraines,
10. presence of hydrocephalus,
11. development of cerebral edema,
12. occurrence of stroke post admission,
13. development of vasospasm during course of treatment,
14. seizures requiring antiepileptic medications

Treatment-Related Neurologic Risk Factors

1. time to surgical treatment (hours),
2. treatment arm,
3. severe vasospasm requiring balloon angioplasty.

The dependent variable used for statistical analysis is the dichotomized Glasgow Outcome Score at three months, that is good or poor outcome. Good outcome represents functional independence (GOS 5 or 4). Poor outcome represents functional dependence (GOS 3), persistent vegetative state (GOS 2) or death (GOS 1).

For the Kurashiki Central Hospital database (n = 504 patients), independent variables include prognostic factors relating to the patients' demographic states, systemic and neurologic risk factors:

Demographic Risk Factors

1. age (in years),
2. sex

Systemic Risk Factors

1. history of hypertension,
2. history of diabetes mellitus,
3. history of blood thinner (antiplatelet or anticoagulant) use,
4. history of heart disease,
5. history of kidney disease,
6. history of liver disease,
7. history of lung disease,
8. history of hospital-acquired infections

Non-Treatment Related Neurologic Risk Factors

1. neurological grade (World Federation of Neurological Surgeons) on admission,
2. aneurysm location (anterior or posterior circulation),
3. aneurysm size (mm),
4. modified Fisher score (thin or thick subarachnoid hemorrhage, along with presence of intraventricular hemorrhage),
5. presence of intraventricular hemorrhage,
6. amount of subarachnoid hemorrhage (score 0-30, based on the Hijdra scale),
7. presence of acute subdural hematoma,
8. presence of intracerebral hemorrhage,
9. presence of delayed stroke,
10. presence of brain swelling,

Treatment-Related Neurologic Risk Factors

1. aneurysm clipping or clipping,
2. seizure requiring antiepileptic medication,
3. chronic hydrocephalus requiring shunting procedure for diversion,
4. presence of stroke (arterial or venous) or rebleeding as complication

The dependent variable captured with the Kurashiki Hospital database was the modified Rankin Score at three months. For analysis, the dichotomized modified Rankin Score at three months was used, where good outcome represents functional independence (mRS 0-3), and poor outcome represents functional dependence (severe disability), vegetative state and death. Using IBM SPSS Version 19.0™, independent variables were entered into univariate models in which chi-square analyses were performed to investigate associations with poor outcome. Two-way interaction terms that included neurologic and systemic prognostic factors were examined. Variables that reached a probability of 0.10 were then entered into a multivariable binary logistic regression model. Variables that reached p value 0.05 were deemed significant. Multivariable analyses had at least 10 subjects per independent variable, which is the minimum number required for a stable multivariable model using logistic regression.

A Priori Hypotheses for Brain-Body Interactions

A priori hypotheses investigated regarding possible interactions between the brain and other organ systems are listed as follows:

Systemic Factors and Rationale for Investigating Brain-Body Interactions

Age

Age, along with clinical pre-operative grade and CT findings are associated with poor neurological outcome in aneurysmal SAH. Both cerebral and systemic atherosclerotic changes occur as one ages.

Hypertension

Hypertension is associated with poor neurological outcome in aneurysmal SAH as it predisposes to hemodynamic related structural damage in cerebral blood vessels, including endothelial damage and decreased elasticity of blood vessel wall.

History of Diabetes

Diabetes and poor glycemic control are associated with symptomatic vasospasm. Insulin resistance is associated with dysfunction of vascular resistance vessels, including endothelial hypertrophy and altered contractile properties.

History of Liver Disease

Hepatic dysfunction is associated with poor clinical grade at hospital admission. During the course of treatment, liver dysfunction is observed in up to 25% of aneurysmal SAH patients.

History of Thyroid Disease

Sick euthyroid syndrome may be observed in aneurysmal SAH patients with previously normal functioning thyroid gland. During acute physiological stress, these patients may have decreased amounts of thyroid hormone, and inhibition of thyroxine production by elevated cortisol levels.

Occurrence of Fever at One Week Post Admission

Fevers are associated with increased cerebral metabolic rates. Even one episode of fever after aneurysmal SAH can be associated with poor outcome.

History of Myocardial Infarction

Patients with a history of myocardial infarction are prone to troponin elevations and decompensated heart failure after SAH. Those with elevated troponin levels and heart failure are more likely to have significant morbidity and mortality.

Neurologic Factors and Specific A Priori Hypotheses

Neurological Grade

We will investigate the degree by which admission neurological grade influences clinical outcome if the aneurysmal SAH patients also have the following conditions, as they are prone to complications arising from them:

1. increasing age (age and neurological grade),
2. hypertension (hypertension and neurological grade),
3. diabetes (diabetes and neurological grade),
4. liver disease (liver disease and neurological grade),
5. thyroid disease (thyroid disease and neurological grade),
6. fever (fever and neurological grade), and
7. myocardial infarction (myocardial infarction and neurological grade).

Occurrence of Stroke Post Admission

We hypothesize that aneurysmal SAH patients who experience post admission stroke may have poor clinical outcome if they also have the following conditions:

1. increasing age (age and stroke),
2. hypertension (hypertension and stroke),
3. diabetes (diabetes and stroke),
4. liver disease (liver disease and stroke),
5. fever (fever and stroke), and
6. myocardial infarction (myocardial infarction and stroke).

Aneurysmal SAH patients with post admission stroke and the aforementioned systemic conditions are predisposed to related complications including rebleeding, seizures, cerebral edema, delayed stroke and vasospasm.

Development of Vasospasm during Course of Treatment

Aneurysmal SAH patients who experience vasospasm may be predisposed to poor clinical outcome as they are more likely to experience complications including delayed stroke and rebleeding if they concomitantly have the following conditions:

1. hypertension (hypertension and vasospasm),
2. diabetes (diabetes and vasospasm),
3. liver disease (liver disease and vasospasm),
4. fever (fever and vasospasm), and
5. myocardial infarction (myocardial infarction and vasospasm).

Seizures Requiring Antiepileptic Medications

We hypothesize that aneurysmal SAH patients with the following systemic conditions who experience seizures may be predisposed to poor clinical outcome arising from complications including status epilepticus, cerebral edema, vasospasm and delayed stroke:

1. increasing age (age and seizures),
2. hypertension (hypertension and seizures),
3. diabetes (diabetes and seizures),
4. liver disease (liver disease and seizures),
5. fever (fever and seizures), and
6. myocardial infarction (myocardial infarction and seizures).

Aneurysm Size

Aneurysmal SAH patients with hypertension (hypertension and aneurysm size) and myocardial infarction (myocardial infarction and aneurysm size) may experience rebleeding complicating their clinical course leading to poor clinical outcome.

Presence of Intraventricular Hemorrhage

We hypothesize that aneurysmal SAH patients with intraventricular hemorrhage and the following systemic conditions are more likely to experience complications including hydrocephalus and rebleeding which may lead to poor clinical outcome:

1. increasing age (age and intraventricular hemorrhage),
2. hypertension (hypertension and intraventricular hemorrhage),
3. diabetes (diabetes and intraventricular hemorrhage),
4. liver disease (liver disease and intraventricular hemorrhage),
5. fever (fever and intraventricular hemorrhage), and
6. myocardial infarction (myocardial infarction and intraventricular hemorrhage).

Presence of Intracerebral Hemorrhage

Aneurysmal SAH patients with post admission intracerebral hemorrhage are prone to poor clinical outcome arising from complications including rebleeding, seizures, cerebral edema and vasospasm, if they also have the following conditions:

1. increasing age (age and intracerebral hemorrhage),
2. hypertension (hypertension and intracerebral hemorrhage),
3. diabetes (diabetes and intracerebral hemorrhage),
4. liver disease (liver disease and intracerebral hemorrhage),
5. fever (fever and intracerebral hemorrhage), and
6. myocardial infarction (myocardial infarction and intracerebral hemorrhage).

Development of Cerebral Edema

We hypothesize that aneurysmal SAH patients who develop post rupture cerebral edema and, concomitantly, have the following conditions, may be prone to poor clinical outcome:

1. increasing age (age and cerebral edema),
2. hypertension (hypertension and cerebral edema),

3. diabetes (diabetes and cerebral edema),
4. liver disease (liver disease and cerebral edema),
5. fever (fever and cerebral edema), and
6. myocardial infarction (myocardial infarction and cerebral edema).

These patients may experience seizures and delayed stroke as possible related complications.

Results

For the Tirilazad and Kurashiki Central Hospital databases, variables and interaction terms that reached a probability of 0.10 were entered into the multivariable binary logistic regression model. These significant single prognostic variables and interaction terms were entered into a multivariable binary logistic regression model. The final models using these databases are illustrated below:

Table 3.2. Statistically significant terms in the final binary logistic regression model using the Tirilazad database

Variable Terms	Odds Ratios	95% Confidence Intervals	p value
Neurological grade (Hunt and Hess)	2.06	1.83-2.32	<0.01
Age (per year)	1.06	1.05-1.07	<0.01
Time to surgery (hour)	1.01	1.00-1.02	0.02
Stroke	4.03	2.11-7.69	<0.01
Seizures by fever on day 8	2.39	1.86-3.06	<0.01
Brain edema by hepatic disease	5.47	1.13-26.46	0.03
Brain edema by hypertension	2.66	1.59-4.45	<0.01
Seizures by myocardial infarction	3.05	1.35-6.87	0.01

Table 3.3. Statistically significant terms in the final binary logistic regression model using the Kurashiki Central Hospital database

Variable Terms	Odds Ratios	95% Confidence Intervals	p value
Neurological grade (WFNS)	1.58	1.32-1.90	<0.01
Age (per year)	1.08	1.05-1.10	<0.01
Complication (Stroke +/- Rebleeding)	25.90	1.46-459.75	0.03
History of heart disease	2.93	1.08-7.97	0.04
History of kidney disease	3.77	1.21-11.72	0.02
History of brain swelling	6.78	1.66-27.79	0.01
History of hydrocephalus requiring shunting procedure	5.34	2.42-11.76	<0.01
Seizures by infection	11.60	1.12-120.67	0.04

Both multivariable binary logistic regression models found three common statistically significant single prognostic variables, namely, admission neurological grade, age and post-admission stroke. The Kurashiki Central Hospital database also found the history of heart disease, kidney disease and hydrocephalus requiring shunt procedure to be statistically significant, while the Tirilazad database found the timing of surgery to be significant.

In terms of interaction terms, both databases found that the odds for predicting poor outcome is increased when the aneurysmal SAH patient experiences fever and infection post hospital admission as well as seizures. The Tirilazad database found that the odds of poor outcome is increased by a factor of 2.39 when the aneurysmal SAH patient experiences fever one week post hospital admission and seizures, while the Kurashiki Central Hospital database found that the odds of poor outcome is increased by a factor of 11.60 when the aneurysmal SAH patient experiences infection post hospital admission and seizures.

In addition, three other statistically significant interaction terms were found in the Tirilazad database, with observations listed as follows:

1. the odds of poor outcome is increased by a factor of 5.47 when the aneurysmal SAH patient with history of hepatic disease develops cerebral edema,
2. the odds of poor outcome is increased by a factor of 2.66 when the aneurysmal SAH patient with history of hypertension develops cerebral edema, and
3. the odds of poor outcome is increased by a factor of 3.05 when the aneurysmal SAH patient with history of myocardial infarction develops seizures.

Discussion

There has been scarce literature to attempt to characterize complex brain-body associations in patients with ruptured brain aneurysms. This analysis included both non-treatment and treatment related prognostic factors, as well as two-way interactions, which described clinically relevant brain-body associations in aneurysmal SAH. The main effects logistic regression models of both databases confirmed the significance of neurological grade, age and stroke in outcome prognosis in aneurysmal SAH.

Seizures

Seizures post aneurysmal SAH increase mortality. The observed incidence of seizures can be as high as 15% in the aneurysmal SAH patient population. The occurrence of seizures in the clinical settings of post admission infection and fever, with a background of myocardial disease, significantly increases morbidity and mortality. Fevers increase cerebral metabolic rate and exacerbate secondary injury, leading to increased risks of delayed strokes. Early onset fevers can be secondary to dysfunction of temperature regulation centers in the hypothalamus whereas late onset fevers are more likely to be infectious, but can include fevers secondary to drug-drug interactions and pulmonary embolism. Exogenous and endogenous pyrogens increase the propensity for fevers and seizure development. In febrile states, inflammatory cytokines increase neuronal excitability via temperature sensitive ion channels leading to increased likelihood of synchronized neuronal activity. Not only is it essential to monitor and treat both seizures and fevers themselves, it is also important to search for underlying etiologies, including infections, pulmonary embolism, drug-drug interactions and delayed strokes which may alter seizure thresholds in the febrile aneurysmal SAH patient.

Our analysis also makes the observation that seizures in the setting of history of myocardial infarction increase the odds of poor outcome. Epilepsy decreases heart rate variability, and is a predictor of sudden cardiac death during seizures with sympathetic overdrive and vagal withdrawal. Ictal tachycardia is more prominent after mesial temporal lobe seizures. Affected epilepsy patients show an increased low frequency component of heart rate variability, reflecting an increased sympathetic modulation of the sinus node, along with decreased parasympathetic activity. Thus, repetitive autonomic stimulation can occur in the actively seizing aneurysmal SAH patient in a lock step phenomenon which can trigger the development of cardiac ictal arrthymias. Continuous cardiac sympathetic discharges and cortical epileptiform activity can occur in a synchronized time-locked manner. These repetitive synchronized autonomic sympathetic discharges lead to cardiac ischemia and structural damage to the myocardium. In aneurysmal SAH patients with pre-existing coronary artery disease and seizures, the propensity of cardiac ischemia is increased, along with potentially fatal multi-systemic complications, including development of neurogenic pulmonary edema and respiratory suppression associated with fatal cardiac tachy- or bradyarrthymias, or cardiac asystole. Multi-system critical care cardiovascular and respiratory supports, therefore, are essential in these epileptic aneurysmal SAH patients in order to maximize their chances of survival.

Hypertension

Hypertension has direct effects of sympathetic nervous system activation and blunting of parasympathetic activity, as reflected with decreased heart rate variability. In the chronic setting, beta adrenergic receptors are upregulated with resetting of the baroreceptor reflex to a higher set point. This altered baroreceptor reflex sensitivity in states of chronic adrenergic stimulation reflects increased sympathetic dominance with upregulation of the renin-angiotensin-aldosterone system. Chronic hypertension is associated with:

1. increased catecholamine secretion,
2. insulin metabolic abnormalities,
3. increased sympathetic outflow to the kidneys with increased renal sodium and water retention, increased renin release, increased endothelin I and angiotensin II production as vasoconstrictors, and
4. decreased nitric oxide mediated endothelial relaxation.

In our two cohorts, we make the observation that development of cerebral edema, in the context of history of hypertension and liver disease, has significant impact on neurologic outcome deterioration in aneurysmal SAH.

By itself, development of cerebral edema may predispose the aneurysmal SAH patient to poor neurological outcome. Further examination of systemic factors revealed that aneurysmal SAH patients with a history of hypertension and development of cerebral edema have 2.7 fold increased odds of poor neurologic outcome. Patients with a history of hypertension are more prone to defective cerebral autoregulation. When cerebral dysautoregulation is present after aneurysmal SAH, brain engorgement can occur as plasma proteins leak from capillaries with increased permeability. Extracellular vasogenic edema may follow as a result of increased hydrostatic pressures, with predilection for posterior cerebral circulation territories. It is important, therefore, to recognize that chronic hypertensive patients have altered elevated blood pressure ranges for autoregulation. It is also essential to monitor for development of cerebral edema in these patients.

This study also makes the novel observation that development of cerebral edema in aneurysmal SAH patients with history of liver dysfunction markedly increases likelihood of poor outcome. Similar to patients with hypertensive history, patients with chronic liver disease have been shown to have altered cerebral autoregulation and cerebral blood flow with decreased cerebral blood flow in the anterior cingulum and increased blood flow in the basal ganglia and occipital lobes at baseline. In acute stages of ruptured cerebral aneurysms, these patients' blood brain barriers become disrupted with marked increased cerebral blood flow secondary to luxury perfusion, thus, predisposing them to development of vasogenic edema. In addition, cytotoxic osmoregulatory mechanisms are involved whereby astrocytes swell secondary to the toxic effects of ammonia and glutamate. The end result is a vicious cycle of neuronal swelling and death, marked increases in cerebral blood flow (cerebral hyperemia) and cerebral edema. It is important, therefore, to prevent development of hepatic encephalopathy and monitor for cerebral edema in aneurysmal SAH patients who have chronic liver dysfunction.

Stroke

Central autonomic network activation can be observed in insular strokes, whereby affected patients showed increased incidences of arrthymias within the first seven days of the event. Stroke patients may exhibit decreased heart rate variability with decreased high and low frequency powers predisposing patients to increased incidences of sudden cardiac death. As a reflection of injury to the baroreflex neural network, baroreceptor sensitivity of the heart, as well as stretch receptors in the aortic arch and carotid sinus show reduced sensitivity, with blunted heart rate changes in response to blood pressure changes. Treatment with beta blockers can decrease the low frequency to high frequency ratio, with shift in sympathovagal balance signaling improved neurologic prognosis.

This current study demonstrates that the odds for predicting poor neurological outcome is increased by a factor of four in aneurysmal SAH patients who develop post-admission strokes. With modern modalities of routine cerebral surveillance imaging over the course of treatment, up to half of aneurysmal SAH patients have observed non-resolving hypodensities, and persistent areas of cerebral perfusion deficits, consistent with stroke. It is increasingly recognized that cerebral infarction after aneurysmal SAH may occur early after aneurysmal rupture or in a delayed manner. Factors associated with development of cerebral infarction include admission neurological status, treatment related complications and occurrence of symptomatic vasospasm. Secondary injury cascade events predisposing aneurysmal SAH patients to post admission strokes include: (1) microthrombi formation, (2) cortical spreading depression, (3) microvasuclar constriction, (4) proliferation of pro-inflammatory cascade, (5) presence of blood-brain barrier disruption, and (6) inadequate collateral circulations.

Conclusion

Our analyses made use of two aneurysmal SAH databases incorporating both multicenter involvement and contemporary advances in the treatment of aneurysmal SAH. Both single prognostic factors and brain-body interactions are explored to make several novel observations which significantly influence clinical outcome in aneurysmal SAH patients. Further studies can be carried out to generalize these observations to other aneurysmal SAH patient populations.

References

[1] Andreasen A, Bartek J, Andresen M, et al. Modifiable risk factors for aneurysmal subarachnoid hemorrhage. *Stroke*. 2013;44(12):3607-12.

[2] Barrett K, Ganong W. *Ganong's review of medical physiology*. New York: McGraw-Hill Medical, 2010.

[3] Bederson J, AANS Publications Committee. *Subarachnoid hemorrhage: pathophysiology and management*. Park Ridge, Ill.: American Association of Neurological Surgeons, 1997.

[4] Butterworth R. The liver-brain axis in liver failure: neuroinflammation and encephalopathy. *Nat Rev Gastroenterol Hepatol*. 2013;10(9):522.

[5] Devinsky O. Effects of seizures on autonomic and cardiovascular function. *Epilepsy Currents*. 2004;4(2):43-46.

[6] Dimopoulou I, Kouyialis A, Tzanella M, et al. High incidence of neuroendocrine dysfunction in long-term survivors of aneurysmal subarachnoid hemorrhage. *Stroke*. 2004;35(12):2884-9.

[7] Dooley J, Sherlock S. *Sherlock's diseases of the liver and biliary system.* Chichester, West Sussex; Hoboken, NJ: Wiley-Blackwell, 2011.

[8] Dube C, Brewster A, Baram T. Febrile seizures: mechanisms and relationship to epilepsy. *Brain and Development*. 2009;31(5):366-71.

[9] Dumont T, Rughani A, Silver J, et al. Diabetes mellitus increases risk of vasospasm following aneurysmal subarachnoid hemorrhage independent of glycemic control. *Neurocrit Care.* 2009;11(2):183-9.

[10] Guyton A, Hall J. *Textbook of medical physiology*. Philadelphia: Saunders, 2000.

[11] Haley EC Jr, Kassell NF, Alves WM, et al. Phase II trial of tirilazad in aneurysmal subarachnoid hemorrhage. A report of the Cooperative Aneurysm Study. *J Neurosurg.* 1995;82:786–90.

[12] Haley EC Jr, Kassell NF, Apperson-Hansen C, et al. A randomized, double-blind, vehicle-controlled trial of tirilazad mesylate in patients with aneurysmal subarachnoid hemorrhage: a cooperative study in North America. *J Neurosurg*. 1997;86:467–74.

[13] Horiuchi T, Tanaka Y, Hongo K. Surgical treatment for aneurysmal subarachnoid hemorrhage in the 8th and 9th decades of life. *Neurosurg.* 2005;56(3):469-75.

[14] Hosmer D, Lemeshow S, Sturdivant R. *Applied logistic regression*. Hoboken, NH: Wiley, 2013.

[15] Ilodigwe D, Gordon M, Kassell N, et al. Sliding dichotomy compared with fixed dichotomization of ordinal outcome scales in subarachnoid hemorrhage trials. *J Neurosurg*. 2013; 118(1), 3-12.

[16] Jang Y, Ilodigwe D, Macdonald R. Metaanalysis of tirilazad mesylate in patients with aneurysmal subarachnoid hemorrhage. *Neurocrit Care*. 2009;10(1):141-7.

[17] Jansen K, Lagae L. Cardiac changes in epilepsy. *Seizure.* 2010;19(8):455-460.

[18] Jennett B, Bond M. Assessment of outcome after severe brain damage: a practical scale. *Lancet.* 1975;480-4.

[19] Kamath M, Watanabe M, Upton ARM. *Heart rate variability (HRV) signal analysis: clinical applications.* Boca Raton: Taylor & Francis, 2013.

[20] Kang J, Shen W, Macdonald R. Why does fever trigger febrile seizures? *J of Neurosci.* 2006;26(9):2590-7.

[21] Kassell N, Haley E, Apperson-Hansen C, Alves W. Randomized, double-blind, vehicle-controlled trial of tirilazad mesylate in patients with aneurysmal subarachnoid hemorrhage: a cooperative study in Europe, Australia and New Zealand. *J Neurosurg.* 1996;84:221-8.

[22] Kim W, Neal L, Hoh B. Risk factors, incidence and effect of cardiac failure and myocardial infarction in aneurysmal subarachnoid hemorrhage patients. *Neurosurg*. 2013;73(3):450-7.

[23] Kumar P, Brown J, Dhar N, et al. Early vs delayed cerebral infarction after aneurysm repair after subarachnoid hemorrhage. *Neurosurg.* 2013;73(4):617-23.

[24] Lannes M, Teitelbaum J, del Pilar Cortes M, Cardoso M, Angle M. Milrinone and homeostasis to treat cerebral vasospasm associated with subarachnoid hemorrhage: the Montreal Neurological Hospital protocol. *Neurocrit Care.* 2012 June;16(3):354-62.

[25] Lanzino G, Kassel N. Double-blind, randomized, vehicle-controlled study of high-dose tirilazad mesylate in women with aneurysmal subarachnoid hemorrhage. Part II. A cooperative study in North America. *J Neurosurg*. 1999;90:1018-24.

[26] Lanzino G, Kassel N, Dorsch N, et al. Double-blind, randomized, vehicle-controlled study of high-dose tirilazad mesylate in women with aneurysmal subarachnoid hemorrhage. Part I. A cooperative

study in Europe, Australia, New Zealand and South Africa. *J Neurosurg.* 1999;90:1011-7.

[27] Layon A, Gabrielli A, Friedman W. *Textbook of neurointensive care.* Philadelphia: Saunders, 2004.

[28] Lee K. *The neuroICU book.* New York: McGraw-Hill Medical, 2012.

[29] Lee V, Oh J, Mulvagh S, et al. Mechanisms in neurogenic stress cardiomyopathy after aneurysmal subarachnoid hemorrhage. *Neurocrit Care.* 2006;5(3):243-9.

[30] Lindekleiv H, Sandvei M, Romundstad P, et al. Joint effect of modifiable risk factors on the risk of aneurysmal subarachnoid hemorrhage: a cohort study. *Stroke.* 2012;43(7):1885-9.

[31] Lo BWY, Fukuda H, Angle M, et al. Clinical outcome prediction in aneurysmal subarachnoid hemorrhage - Alterations in brain-body interface. *Surg Neurol Int.* 2016 Aug 1;7(Suppl 18):S527-37.

[32] Lo BWY, Fukuda H, Angle M, et al. Aneurysmal subarachnoid hemorrhage prognostic decision-making algorithm using classification and regression tree analysis. *Surg Neurol Int.* 2016 Jul 7;7:73.

[33] Lo BWY, Fukuda H, Nishimura Y, et al. *Brain-body interactions: contemporary outcome prediction in aneurysmal subarachnoid hemorrhage using bayesian neural networks and fuzzy logic.* New York: Nova Biomedical, 2014.

[34] Lo BWY, Fukuda H, Nishimura Y, et al. Pathophysiologic mechanisms of brain-body associations in ruptured brain aneurysms: A systematic review. *Surg Neurol Int.* 2015 Aug 11;6:136.

[35] Lo B, Macdonald R, Baker A, et al. Clinical outcome prediction in aneurysmal subarachnoid hemorrhage using Bayesian neural networks with fuzzy logic inferences. *Comput Math Methods* Med. 2013:904860.

[36] Lo B, Nishimura Y, Fukuda H. Clinical outcome prediction using Bayesian regression and artificial neural networks. *Horizons in Neurosciences Research,* Volume 15. New York: NOVA Science Publishers, 2014.

[37] Mangieri P, Suzuki K, Ferreira M, et al. Evaluation of pituitary and thyroid hormones in patients with subarachnoid hemorrhage due to ruptured intracranial aneurysm. *Neuro-Psiquiatr.* 2003;61(1):14.

[38] Mazarati A. Cytokines: a link between fever and seizures. *Epilepsy Currents*. 2005;5(5):169-70.

[39] Mrozek S, Vardon F, Geeraerts T. Brain temperature: physiology and pathophysiology after brain injury. *Anesthesiol Res Pract.* E pub 2012 Dec 26.

[40] O'Carroll R, Ebmeier K, Dougall N, et al. Regional cerebral blood flow and cognitive function in patients with chronic liver disease. *Lancet.* 1991;337(8752):1250-1253.

[41] Olivier D, Arnaud D, Roover P, et al. Brain edema and intracranial hypertension in fulminant hepatic failure. *World Journal of Gastroenterology.* 2006;12(46):7405-7412.

[42] Park J, Woo H, Kang D, et al. Formal protocol for emergency treatment of ruptured intracranial aneurysms to reduce in-hospital rebleeding and improve clinical outcomes. *J Neurosurg*. E pub Nov 18, 2014.

[43] Payen J, Fauvage B, Falcon D, et al. Oedème cérébral par lésion de la barrière hématoencéphalique: mécanismes et diagnostic. [Cerebral edema by lesion of the blood-brain barrier: mechanisms and diagnosis.] *Annales françaises d'anesthesie et de reanimation*: 2003;2(3):220-225.

[44] Rowland L, Pedley T, Merritt H. *Merritt's neurology.* Philadelphia, PA: Lippincott Williams & Wilkins, 2010.

[45] Rowland M, Hadjipavlou G, Kelly M, et al. Delayed cerebral ischaemia after subarachnoid haemorrhage: looking beyond vasospasm. *British Journal of Anaesthesia*. 2012;109(3):315-29.

[46] Sadamasa N, Koyanagi M, Fukuda H, et al. Is aneurysm repair justified for the patients aged 80 or older after aneurysmal subarachnoid hemorrhage? *J Neurointerv Surg*. 2014;6(9),664.

[47] Schneider H, Kreitschmann-Andermahr I, et al. Hypothalamopituitary dysfunction following traumatic brain injury and aneurysmal subarachnoid hemorrhage: a systematic review. *JAMA*. 2007 Sep 26;298(12):1429-38.

[48] Steyerberg E, Vickers A, Cook N, et al. Assessing the performance of prediction models: a framework for traditional and novel measures. *Epidemiol.* 2010;21(1):128-38.

[49] Todd M, Hindman B, Clarke W, et al. Perioperative fever and outcome in surgical patients with aneurysmal subarachnoid hemorrhage. *Neurosurg*. 2009;64(5):897-908.

[50] Torbey M. *Neurocritical care*. Cambridge; New York: Cambridge University Press, 2010.

[51] Varelas P. *Seizures in critical care: a guide to diagnosis and therapeutics.* Totowa, NJ: Humana Press, 2005.

[52] Wijdicks E. *The practice of emergency and critical care neurology*. New Work: Oxford University Press, 2010.

[53] Zhang S, Wang L, Liu M, et al. Tirilazad for aneurysmal subarachnoid hemorrhage (Review). *Cochrane Database Syst Rev.* 2010 Feb 17.

Section Four

Aneurysmal Subarachnoid Hemorrhage Prognostic Decision-Making Algorithms – Comparative Analyses in Two Cohorts

Benjamin W. Y. Lo[1,*], Hitoshi Fukuda[2], Masaomi Koyanagi[3], Adrian Upton[4] and Mitchell A. H. Levine[5]

[1]Departments of Neurosurgery, Neurology and Critical Care Medicine, Montreal Neurological Institute and Hospital, McGill University, Montreal, Canada

[2]Department of Neurosurgery, Kochi University Hospital, Kochi, Japan

[3]Department of Neurosurgery, National Hospital Organization Himeji Medical Center, Himeji, Japan

[*] Corresponding Author Email: benjamin.lo@mcgill.ca.

[4]Division of Neurology, Department of Medicine,
McMaster University, Hamilton, Ontario, Canada
[5]Department of Clinical Epidemiology and Biostatistics
(Department of Health Research Methods, Evidence and Impact),
Department of Medicine, Division of Clinical Pharmacology,
Centre for Evaluation of Medicines, St. Joseph's Hospital,
McMaster University, Hamilton, Ontario, Canada

Introduction

The goal of this section is to use the classification and regression tree analysis technique to create a prognostic decision-making algorithm for aneurysmal SAH. This technique is applied to two patient cohorts, namely, the multicenter Tirilazad database (3551 patients) and a contemporary database from Kurashiki Central Hospital, a stroke center affiliated with Kyoto University, Japan (504 patients). Comparative analysis is conducted to elucidate prognostic subgroups in aneurysmal SAH, taking into account neurologic, systemic and demographic factors. For bedside prognostication and clinical decision-making, a prediction tool can be regarded as a useful adjunct to complement clinical opinion and judgment.

Classification and regression tree analysis is a statistical technique that involves creation of a decision tree by recursive partitioning of a dataset into more homogeneous subgroups. At each node, the best possible split for each variable is found by minimizing the impurity of subsequent daughter nodes. This technique prevents overfitting by pruning terminal nodes or leaves, such that a decision tree is found with the smallest error rates. In addition, model performance can be enhanced by split sample validation techniques. Classification and regression tree analysis is a statistical technique that takes into account non-linear and high order interactions. It can handle large datasets with missing data, as well as high dimensionality.

Methods

The Tirilazad and Kurashiki Central Hospital databases were used to investigate prognostic subgroups for outcome prediction in aneurysmal SAH patients. Descriptions of these databases were given in the previous section. IBM SPSS Version 23.0™ was used to create the CART decision trees.

For the Tirilazad dataset, candidate predictors included independent variables that reached a probability of 0.10 in univariate logistic regression analysis. They include:

1. hospital admission neurological (Hunt and Hess) grade,
2. age (years),
3. time to surgery (hours),
4. occurrence of post admission fever on day 8,
5. aneurysm size (≤ 12 mm or > 12 mm),
6. presence of angiographic vasospasm on hospital admission,
7. presence of intraventricular hemorrhage,
8. development of cerebral edema,
9. presence of intracerebral hemorrhage,
10. history of hypertension,
11. history of myocardial infarction,
12. occurrence of stroke post admission,
13. prior episode of SAH,
14. location of aneurysm,
15. development of vasospasm during course of treatment, and
16. development of seizures requiring antiepileptic medications.

The dependent variable captured with the Tirilazad database was the Glasgow Outcome Score at three months. For analysis, the dichotomized Glasgow Outcome Score at three months was used, where good outcome represents functional independence (GOS 5 and 4), and poor outcome represents functional dependence (GOS 3), persistent vegetative state (GOS 2) or death (GOS 1).

For the Kurashiki Central Hospital database (n = 504 patients), independent variables include prognostic factors relating to the patients' demographic states, systemic and neurologic risk factors:

Demographic Risk Factors

1. age (years),
2. sex

Systemic Risk Factors

1. history of hypertension,
2. history of diabetes mellitus,
3. history of blood thinner (antiplatelet or anticoagulant) use,
4. history of heart disease,
5. history of kidney disease,
6. history of liver disease,
7. history of lung disease,
8. history of hospital-acquired infections

Non-Treatment Related Neurologic Risk Factors

1. neurological grade (World Federation of Neurological Surgeons) on admission,

2. aneurysm location (anterior or posterior circulation),
3. aneurysm size (mm),
4. modified Fisher score (thin or thick subarachnoid hemorrhage, along with presence of intraventricular hemorrhage),
5. presence of intraventricular hemorrhage,
6. amount of subarachnoid hemorrhage (score 0-30, based on the Hijdra scale),
7. presence of acute subdural hematoma,
8. presence of intracerebral hemorrhage,
9. presence of delayed stroke,
10. presence of brain swelling

Treatment Related Neurologic Risk Factors

1. aneurysm clipping or coiling,
2. seizure requiring antiepileptic medications,
3. chronic hydrocephalus requiring shunting procedure for diversion,
4. presence of stroke (arterial or venous) or rebleeding as complication.

The dependent variable captured with the Kurashiki Hospital database was the modified Rankin Score at three months. For analysis, the dichotomized modified Rankin Score at three months was used, where good outcome represents functional independence (mRS 0-3), and poor outcome represents functional dependence (severe disability), vegetative state and death. For both databases, statistical power was ensured by having effective sample size of more than 10 events per variable, with at least 10 patients per final subgroup. For decision tree growing, the Gini index splitting rule was used to decreased variance between classes through reduction of entropy where the largest categories were split into separate subgroups. Overfitting was avoided by using tree pruning. Decision trees were generated with training and testing datasets, with percentages of favorable outcome reported in each terminal prognostic subgroup. Split sample analysis (70% training and 30% testing) was used to examine model performance, with reports of classification accuracy, risk estimate and standard error for each decision tree. Univariate models using chi-square analyses were performed to investigate the associations between explanatory variables generated in the classification trees.

Classification and Regression Tree Analysis Results

In the Tirilazad patient populations, unfavorable outcome (functional dependence, persistent vegetative state and death) at three months after aneurysmal SAH was observed in 1061 (30%) of patients. Classification trees describing the relationships between neurological outcome and explanatory factors in aneurysmal SAH were generated using the training dataset (Figure 4.1) and testing dataset (Figure 4.2). Figures 4.1 and 4.2 demonstrated seven terminal prognostic subgroups with the same node ranking order according to percentages of unfavorable outcomes, with percentage differences between the two decision trees ranging from 1.3 to 7.8%. Seven terminal prognostic subgroups are illustrated as follows:

1. good admission neurological grade (Hunt and Hess grades 1 or 2), absent post-admission stroke (Node #3) – 8.7% unfavorable outcome (training dataset) and 7.4% unfavorable outcome (testing dataset),
2. poor admission neurological grades (Hunt and Hess grades 3 or 4), absent post-admission stroke, absent post-admission fever

(Node #10) – 33.6% unfavorable outcome (training dataset) and 37.4% unfavorable outcome (testing dataset),

3. good admission neurological grades, post-admission stroke, age < 58.5 years (Node #7) – 38.3% unfavorable outcome (training dataset) and 43.8% unfavorable outcome (testing dataset),
4. poor admission neurological grades, absent post-admission stroke, development of post-admission fever (Node #12) – 44.6% unfavorable outcome (training dataset) and 48.6% unfavorable outcome (testing dataset),
5. good admission neurological grades, post-admission stroke, age > 58.5 years (Node #8) – 59.4% unfavorable outcome (training dataset) and 54.7% unfavorable outcome (testing dataset),
6. poor admission neurological grade (Hunt and Hess grade 5), absent post-admission stroke, development of post-admission fever (Node #11) – 69.7% unfavorable outcome (training dataset) and 61.9% unfavorable outcome (testing dataset), and
7. poor admission neurological grades, post-admission stroke (Node #6) – 75.4% unfavorable outcome (training dataset) and 72.9% unfavorable outcome (testing dataset).

The classification and regression tree model generated using the training dataset had a classification accuracy of 79%, risk estimate of 0.21 with standard error of 0.008. The model generated using the testing dataset had a classification accuracy of 77%, risk estimate of 0.23 and standard error of 0.01. The occurrence of fever at one week post-aneurysmal rupture is associated with increased odds of post admission stroke (OR 1.83, 95% CI 1.56-2.45, $p<0.01$). Table 4.1 shows a clinical prognostic decision-making algorithm for aneurysmal subarachnoid hemorrhage patients with prognostic subgroups based on the classification and regression tree derived from the Tirilazad database.

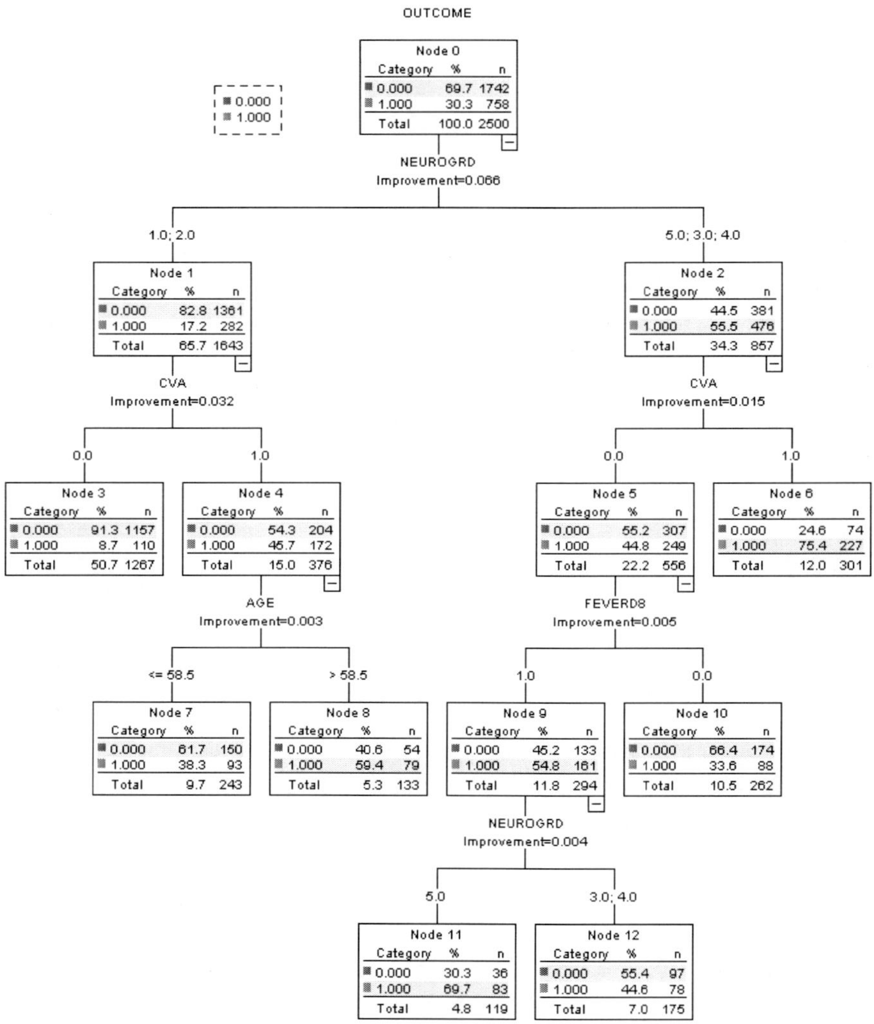

Figure 4.1. Aneurysmal subarachnoid hemorrhage classification tree using training data set (Tirilazad database).

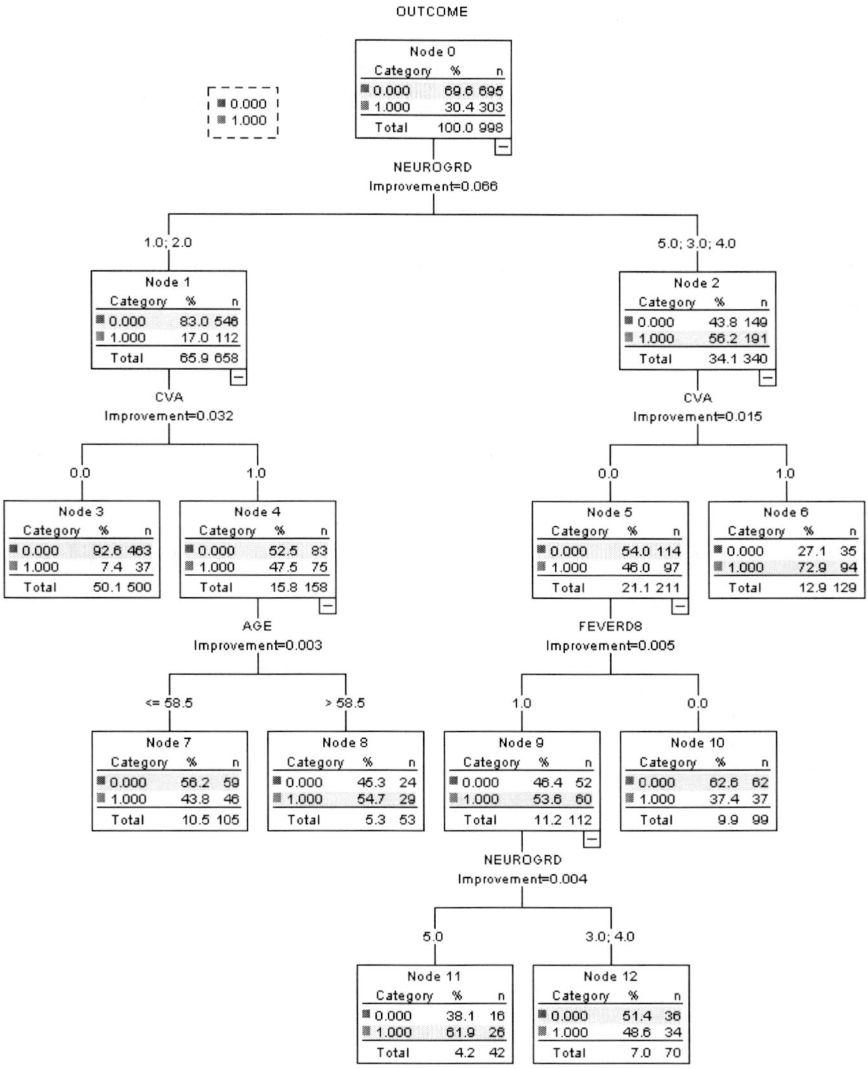

Figure 4.2. Aneurysmal subarachnoid hemorrhage classification tree using testing data set (Tirilazad database).

Table 4.1. Clinical prognostic decision-making algorithm in aneurysmal subarachnoid hemorrhage, with prognostic subgroups based on classification and regression tree derived from the Tirilazad database

Admission neurological grade	Age = 58.5 years	Post-admission fever	Post-admission stroke	Unfavorable outcome (%)	
Poor	Older	Present	Present	75.9%	>75% very high
Poor	Older	Absent	Present	73.6%	50-75% high
Poor	Younger	Present	Present	66.9%	
Good	Older	Present	Present	63.2%	
Poor	Older	Present	Absent	56.6%	
Poor	Younger	Absent	Present	55.4%	
Good	Older	Absent	Present	44.0%	25-50% inter-mediate
Poor	Older	Absent	Absent	41.5%	
Good	Younger	Present	Present	39.0%	
Poor	Younger	Present	Absent	39.0%	
Good	Younger	Absent	Present	25.7%	
Good	Older	Present	Absent	18.5%	<25% low
Poor	Younger	Absent	Absent	17.4%	
Good	Older	Absent	Absent	14.3%	
Good	Younger	Present	Absent	7.9%	
Good	Younger	Absent	Absent	2.0%	

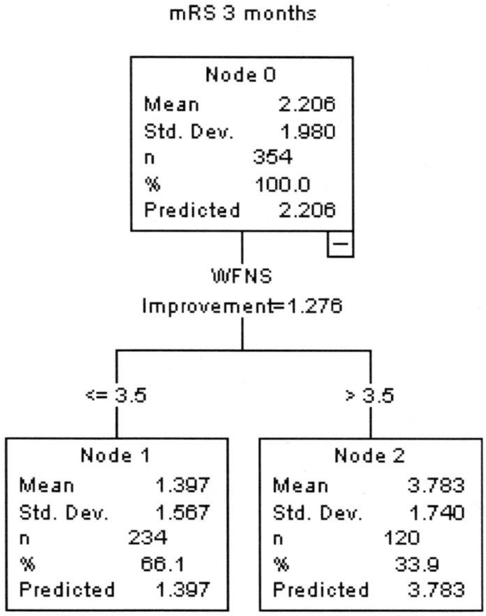

Figure 4.3. Aneurysmal subarachnoid hemorrhage classification tree using training data set (Kurashiki Central Hospital database).

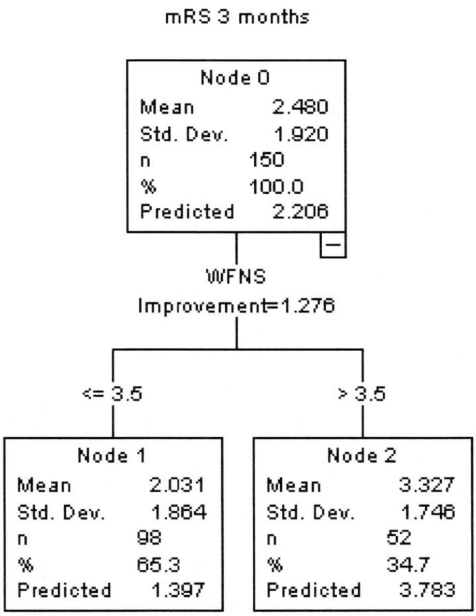

Figure 4.4. Aneurysmal subarachnoid hemorrhage classification tree using testing data set (Kurashiki Central Hospital database).

The Kurashiki Central Hospital database represents our external validation cohort. In this population, unfavorable outcome (severe disability, vegetative state and death) at three months after aneurysmal SAH was observed in 159 (31.5%) of patients. Classification trees describing the relationships between neurological outcome and explanatory factors in aneurysmal SAH were generated using the training dataset (Figure 4.3) and testing dataset (Figure 4.4). Figures 4.3 and 4-4 demonstrated two terminal prognostic subgroups with admission neurological grades (WFNS grades 1, 2, or 3) predicting favorable outcome (training dataset – 66.1% favorable outcome, testing dataset – 65.3% favorable outcome).

Discussion

Clinical prediction tools facilitate the process of prognostication and clinical decision-making for both clinicians and patient families. The current classification and regression tree has seven terminal prognostic subgroups and makes use of the two most frequently retained clinical prognostic factors for long-term neurologic outcome, namely, neurological grade and age. It also demonstrates the significance of both post-admission stroke and fever in outcome prediction. Our external validation cohort confirms the traditional clinical prognostic factor of neurological grade. In the present study, the occurrence of post-admission stroke increases the proportion of unfavorable neurologic outcome in aneurysmal SAH patients originally presenting with favorable admission neurological grades by 30%. In our prior analysis of the Tirilazad database, multivariable logistic regression analysis demonstrated that post-admission stroke increases the odds of poor neurological outcome in aneurysmal SAH patients by four fold (OR 4.03, 95% CI 2.11-7.69, $p<0.01$) [refer to previous section]. Patients experiencing vasospasm are at increased risk of post-admission strokes. Additionally, several secondary injury cascade events may predispose these patients to post-admission strokes, including: (1) microthrombi formation, (2) cortical spreading depression, (3) microvascular constriction, (4) proliferation of pro-inflammatory cascade, (5) presence of blood-brain barrier disruption, and (6) inadequate collateral circulation. Several contemporary neurocritical care strategies are used to decrease the likelihood of post-admission strokes. They include: (1) use of milrinone, an inotropic vasodilator with anti-inflammatory properties, to prevent and treat vasospasm, (2) early decompressive craniectomy in patients with refractory increased intracranial pressures associated with cerebral edema, and (3) monitoring and treating seizures.

Fever is often a clinical indicator of neurological deterioration, as it also triggers events in the secondary cascade of neurological injury. The epileptic aneurysmal SAH patient who develops post-admission fever has an increased odds of poor outcome by a factor of 2.4 (OR 2.4, 95% CI 1.86-3.06, $p<0.01$) [refer to previous section]. The various causes of post-admission late onset fevers, including nosocomial infections, central neurological injury, thromboembolic events and drug-drug interactions, can also lead to neurological complications, including increased intracranial pressures, cerebral edema and post-admission strokes. The occurrence of fever at one week post hospital admission is associated with increased odds of post admission strokes (OR 1.83, 95% CI 1.56-2.15, $p<0.01$), including vasospasm-induced delayed strokes. Aggressive symptomatic control and rigorous search for underlying etiology are, therefore, warranted.

Conclusion

Clinical outcome after aneurysmal SAH may be influenced by interactions among a number of brain-body associations. Classification tree algorithm serves as a useful tool for prognostic decision-making. The prognostic subgroups demonstrated the interplay of various underlying pathophysiologic mechanisms which, together, may adversely influence long-term neurologic outcome after aneurysmal SAH.

The classification tree generated in this chapter increases clinician and patient family awareness of the various demographic, neurologic and systemic prognostic factors which are pertinent for initial prognostication, namely, admission neurological grade and patient age. It also alerts the clinician to two important brain-body associations, including the occurrence of fever and delayed strokes, which may arise during hospitalization severely affecting patient outcomes. The clinician is, then, encouraged to tailor various treatment efforts to prevent and treat these, as well as other alterations in the brain-body interface in order to maximize the chances of survival and recovery after aneurysmal subarachnoid hemorrhage.

References

[1] Breiman L. *Classification and regression trees*. Belmont, CA: Wadsworth, 1984.

[2] De'ath G, Fabricius K. Classification and regression trees: a powerful yet simple technique for ecological data analysis. *Ecology* 2000(81):3178-92.

[3] Germanson T, Lanzino G, Kongable G, Torner J, Kassell N. Risk classification after aneurysmal subarachnoid hemorrhage. *Surg Neurol* 1998;49:155-63.

[4] Kahn J, Caldwell E, Deem S, Newell D, Heckbert S, Rubenfeld G. Acute lung injury in patients with subarachnoid hemorrhage: incidence, risk factors and outcome. *Crit Care Med* 2006;34:196-202.

[5] Karamanakos P, von Und Zu Fraunberg M, Bendel S, et al. Risk factors for three phases of 12-month mortality in 1657 patients from a defined population after acute aneurysmal subarachnoid hemorrhage. *World Neurosurg* 2012;78:631-9.

[6] Lo B, Stojic F, Spears J, Schweizer T, Macdonald R. Clinical outcomes, stroke trials and cognitive outcome. In *The Behavioral Consequences of Stroke*. (pp. 283-314). New York: Springer, 2014.

[7] Lo B, Fukuda H. Pathophysiology of brain somatic interactions in aneurysmal subarachnoid hemorrhage – review and update. *Brain Disord Ther* 2015;4:183.

[8] Lo B, Fukuda H, Nishimura Y, et al. Systematic review of clinical prediction tools and prognostic factors in aneurysmal subarachnoid hemorrhage. *Surg Neurol Int* 2015;6:135.

[9] Lo B, Fukuda H, Nishimura Y, et al. Pathophysiologic mechanisms of brain-body associations in ruptured brain aneurysms: a systematic review. *Surg Neurol Int* 2015;6:136.

[10] McGirt M, Woodworth G, Ali M, et al. Persistent perioperative hyperglycemia as an independent predictor of poor outcome after aneurysmal subarachnoid hemorrhage. *J Neurosurg* 2007; 107:1080-5.

[11] Moisen G. Classification and regression trees. In *Encyclopedia of Ecology*. (pp 582-88). Oxford, UK: Elsevier, 2008.

[12] Ogilvy C, Cheung A, Mitha A, et al. Outcomes for surgical and endovascular management of intracranial aneurysms using a comprehensive grading system. *Neurosurg* 2006;59:1037-42.

[13] Rabinstein A, Friedman J, Nichols D, et al. Predictors of outcome after endovascular treatment of cerebral vasospasm. *AJNR* 2004;25:1778-82.

[14] Risselada R, Lingsma H, Bauer-Mehren A, et al. Prediction of 60 day case-fatality after aneurysmal subarachnoid haemorrhage:

results from the International Subarachnoid Aneurysm Trial (ISAT). *Eur J Epidemiol* 2010;25:261-6.

[15] Rosengart A, Schultheiss K, Tolentino J, et al. Prognostic factors for outcome in patients with aneurysmal subarachnoid hemorrhage. *Stroke* 2007;38:2315-21.

[16] Sanchez C, Ogilvy C, Carter B. Outcomes studies in cerebrovascular neurosurgery. *Neurosurg Focus* 2007;22(3):E11.

[17] Yohannes Y, Webb P. *Classification and regression trees, CART: a user manual for identifying indicators of vulnerability to famine and chronic food insecurity*. Washington, D.C.: International Food Policy Research Institute, 1999.

Section Five

The Brain-Body Interface in Aneurysmal Subarachnoid Hemorrhage – Exploratory Analyses Using Artificial Neural Networks

Benjamin W. Y. Lo[1,*], Hitoshi Fukuda[2], Masaomi Koyanagi[3], Benedict Taw[4], Matthew Wai-Man Lui[4], Hidetoshi Kasuya[5], Adrian Upton[6] and Mitchell A. H. Levine[7]

[1]Departments of Neurosurgery, Neurology and Critical Care Medicine, Montreal Neurological Institute and Hospital, McGill University, Montreal, Canada

[2]Department of Neurosurgery, Kochi University Hospital, Kochi, Japan

[*] Corresponding Author Email: benjamin.lo@mcgill.ca.

[3]Department of Neurosurgery,
National Hospital Organization Himeji Medical Center,
Himeji, Japan
[4]Division of Neurosurgery, Queen Mary Hospital,
University of Hong Kong, Hong Kong
[5]Department of Neurosurgery,
Tokyo Women's Medical University Medical Center East,
Tokyo, Japan
[6]Division of Neurology, Department of Medicine,
McMaster University, Hamilton, Ontario, Canada
[7]Department of Clinical Epidemiology and Biostatistics
(Department of Health Research Methods, Evidence and Impact),
Department of Medicine, Division of Clinical Pharmacology,
Centre for Evaluation of Medicines, St. Joseph's Hospital,
McMaster University, Hamilton, Ontario, Canada

Introduction

The goal of this section is to use artificial neural networks for exploratory analyses to further characterize brain-body interactions among neurologic, systemic and demographic prognostic factors in aneurysmal SAH. This technique is applied to two patient cohorts, namely, the multicenter Tirilazad database (3551 patients) and a contemporary database from Kurashiki Central Hospital, a stroke center affiliated with Kyoto University, Japan (504 patients).

Artificial neural networks are intelligent systems that take into account both linear and complex non-linear complex relationships among measured and latent (unobservable) variables. They can learn and change behaviour as they gain experience and store knowledge using internodal connection strengths known as synaptic weights.

Optimization processes are carried out to minimize error functions (differences between predicted and actual outcome values). More detailed discussion of artificial neural network theories can be found with this book's companion "Brain-Body Interactions – Contemporary Outcome Prediction in Aneurysmal Subarachnoid Hemorrhage using Bayesian Neural Networks and Fuzzy Logic."

Methods

The Tirilazad and Kurashiki Central Hospital databases were used for artificial neural network analyses in aneurysmal SAH patient cohorts. Descriptions of these databases were given in Section Three. IBM SPSS Version 23.0™ was used to create the artificial neural network models.

Independent variables recorded in the Tirilizad database are listed as follows:

Demographic Risk Factors

1. age (in years),
2. sex,
3. patient's weight (kg)

Systemic Risk Factors

1. systolic blood pressure (mmHg),
2. diastolic blood pressure (mmHg),
3. temperature on admission (degree Celsius),

4. occurrence of fever one week after hospital admission,
5. history of hypertension,
6. history of angina,
7. history of myocardial infarction,
8. history of diabetes mellitus,
9. history of hepatic disease,
10. history of thyroid disease,
11. development of pulmonary edema

Non-Treatment Related Neurologic Risk Factors

1. hospital admission neurological grade (Hunt and Hess) [1 – asymptomatic, 2 – headaches, cranial nerve palsy, 3 – mild focal deficit, confusion, 4 – stupor, moderate to severe hemiparesis, 5 – deep coma, moribund],
2. aneurysm size (≤ 12 mm or > 12 mm),
3. presence of angiographic vasospasm on hospital admission,
4. presence of intraventricular hemorrhage,
5. presence of intracerebral hemorrhage,
6. location of aneurysm (anterior or posterior circulation),
7. thickness of subarachnoid hemorrhage (≤ 1 mm or > 1 mm),
8. prior episode of subarachnoid hemorrhage,
9. history of migraines,
10. presence of hydrocephalus,
11. development of cerebral edema,
12. occurrence of stroke post admission,
13. development of vasospasm during course of treatment,
14. seizures requiring antiepileptic medications

Treatment-Related Neurologic Risk Factors

1. time to surgical treatment (hours),
2. treatment arm,
3. severe vasospasm requiring balloon angioplasty.

The dependent variable used for statistical analysis is the dichotomized Glasgow Outcome Score at three months, which is good or poor outcome. Good outcome represents functional independence (GOS 5 or 4). Poor outcome represents functional dependence (GOS 3), persistent vegetative state (GOS 2) or death (GOS 1).

For the Kurashiki Central Hospital database (n = 504 patients), independent variables include prognostic factors relating to the patients' demographic states, systemic and neurologic risk factors:

Demographic Risk Factors

1. age (in years),
2. sex

Systemic Risk Factors

1. history of hypertension,
2. history of diabetes mellitus,
3. history of blood thinner (antiplatelet or anticoagulant) use,
4. history of heart disease,
5. history of kidney disease,
6. history of liver disease,
7. history of lung disease,

8. history of hospital-acquired infections

Non-Treatment Related Neurologic Risk Factors

1. neurological grade (World Federation of Neurological Surgeons) on admission,
2. aneurysm location (anterior or posterior circulation),
3. aneurysm size (mm),
4. modified Fisher score (thin or thick subarachnoid hemorrhage, along with presence of intraventricular hemorrhage),
5. presence of intraventricular hemorrhage,
6. amount of subarachnoid hemorrhage (score 0-30, based on the Hijdra scale),
7. presence of acute subdural hematoma,
8. presence of intracerebral hemorrhage,
9. presence of delayed stroke,
10. presence of brain swelling

Treatment-Related Neurologic Risk Factors

1. aneurysm clipping or clipping,
2. seizure requiring antiepileptic medication,
3. chronic hydrocephalus requiring shunting procedure for diversion,
4. presence of stroke (arterial or venous) or rebleeding as complication

The dependent variable captured with the Kurashiki Hospital database was the modified Rankin Score at three months. For analysis, the dichotomized modified Rankin Score at three months was used, where good outcome represents functional independence (mRS 0-3), and poor outcome represents functional dependence (severe disability), vegetative state and death.To explore clinical prognostic factors for aneurysmal subarachnoid hemorrhage, artificial neural networks models were created using IBM SPSS Version 23.0™. Split sample validation technique using 3 partitions (60% training, 20% testing, 20% holdout), and model discrimination were examined. The most robust clinical prediction models were found with estimates of the relative importance of each prognostic variable.

Results

Artificial Neural Networks using the Tirilazad Database

Using the Tirilazad database, the most robust artificial neural networks for clinical prediction in aneurysmal subarachnoid hemorrhage was found using the multilayer perceptron model with 3 partitions (training sample 60%, testing sample 20%, holdout sample 20%), as shown in Figure 5.1.

The network architecture had 1 hidden layer and 10 latent variables. The sigmoid function was specified as the activation function from input to hidden layers, and from hidden to output layers. Training criteria made use of periodic synaptic weight optimization, with the error optimization function using gradient descent.

Training time required 53 seconds. Model classification showed 84% correct predictions in the training sample, 81% correct predictions in the testing sample and 85% correct predictions in the holdout sample. C statistic was used to examine discrimination, with area under the ROC curve being 0.870, for both favorable and unfavorable outcomes (Figure 5.2).

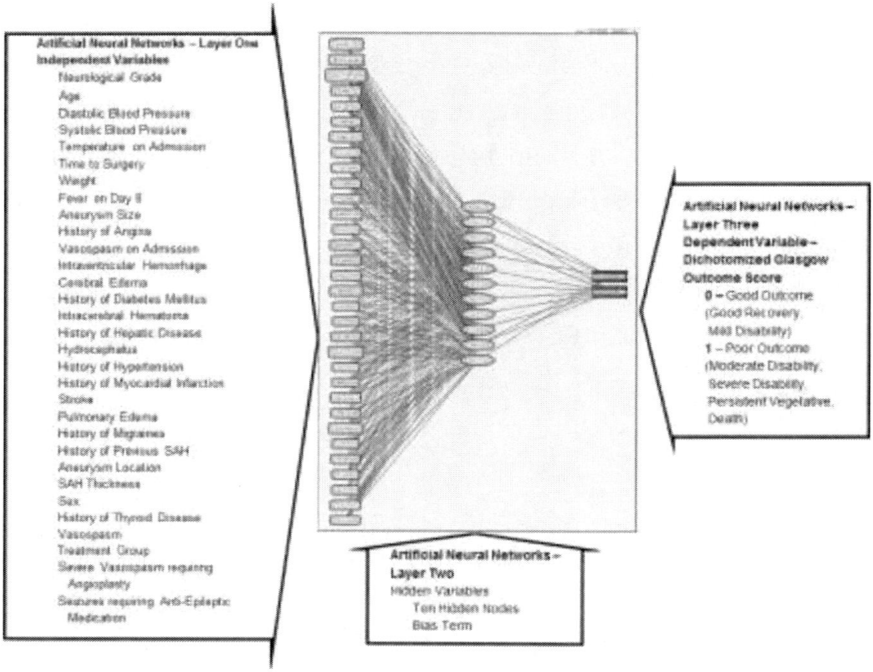

Figure 5.1. Artificial neural networks output using the dichotomized Glasgow Outcome Score with insets for each layer. Output figure generated by IBM SPSS Version 23.0™ (Armonk, NY).

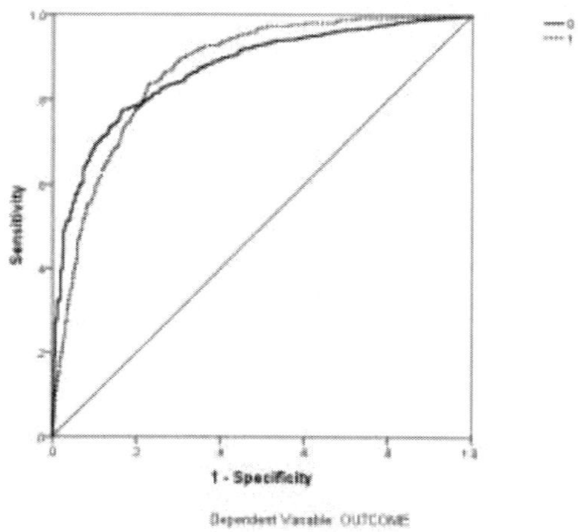

Figure 5.2. ROC curve to analyze model performance. Output figure generated by IBM SPSS Version 23.0™ (Armonk, NY).

Variables in order of magnitude of relative importance are shown as follows:

1. age - 0.132,
2. neurological grade - 0.082,
3. occurrence of stroke post admission - 0.079,
4. thickness of subarachnoid hemorrhage - 0.069,
5. time to surgical treatment - 0.060,
6. history of hepatic disease - 0.054,
7. development of cerebral edema - 0.049,
8. presence of angiographic vasospasm on admission - 0.044,
9. diastolic blood pressure - 0.038,
10. development of severe vasospasm requiring angioplasty - 0.034,
11. presence of previous episode of subarachnoid hemorrhage - 0.032,
12. history of diabetes mellitus - 0.028,
13. temperature on admission - 0.027,
14. presence of intracerebral hematoma on admission - 0.027,
15. presence of fever one week post admission - 0.026,
16. development of seizures requiring use of anti-epileptic medications - 0.025,
17. history of myocardial infarction - 0.024,
18. aneurysm size - 0.023,
19. patient's weight - 0.021,
20. systolic blood pressure on admission - 0.021,
21. history of thyroid disease - 0.019,
22. location of aneurysm - 0.018,
23. history of angina - 0.014,
24. presence of intraventricular hemorrhage on admission - 0.011,
25. history of migraines - 0.009,
26. treatment group - 0.008,
27. development of vasospasm during course of treatment - 0.007,

28. development of pulmonary edema post admission - 0.006,
29. history of hypertension - 0.006,
30. sex - 0.006, and
31. development of hydrocephalus - 0.004.

Artificial Neural Networks using the Kurashiki Central Hospital Database

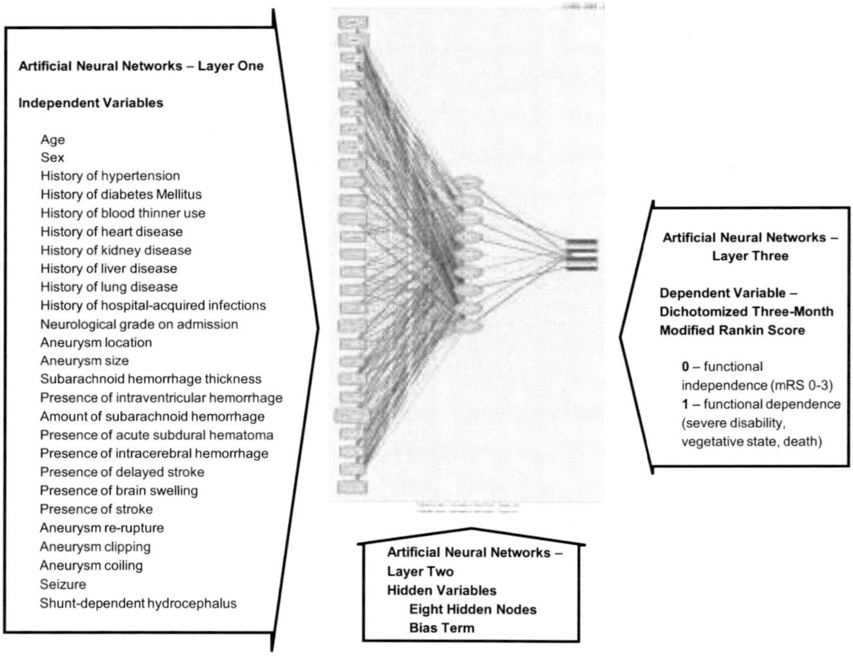

Figure 5.3. Artificial neural networks output using the dichotomized Glasgow Outcome Score with insets for each layer. Output figure generated by IBM SPSS Version 23.0™ (Armonk, NY).

Using the Kurashiki Central Hospital database, the most robust artificial neural networks for clinical prediction in aneurysmal subarachnoid hemorrhage was found using the multilayer perceptron model with 3 partitions (training sample 60%, testing sample 20%, holdout sample 20%), as shown in Figure 5.3.

The network architecture had 1 hidden layer and 8 latent variables. The sigmoid function was specified as the activation function from input to hidden layers, and from hidden to output layers. Training criteria made use of periodic synaptic weight optimization, with the error optimization function using gradient descent.

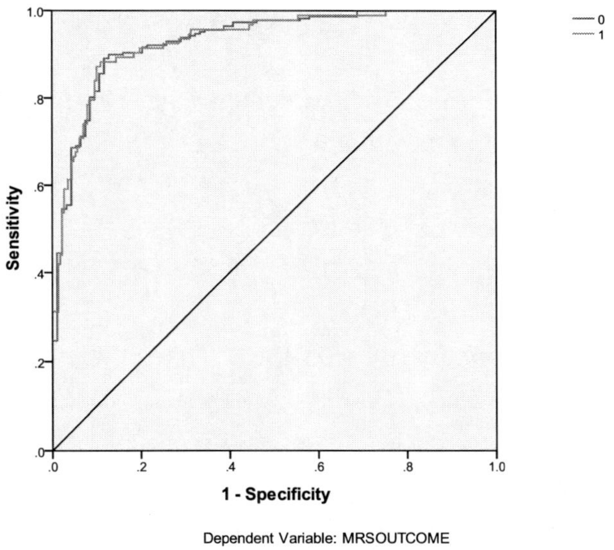

Figure 5.4. ROC curve to analyze model performance. Output figure generated by IBM SPSS Version 23.0™ (Armonk, NY).

Variables in order of magnitude of relative importance are shown as follows:

1. aneurysmal re-rupture – 0.149,
2. age – 0.089
3. hydrocephalus requiring shunt insertion – 0.072,
4. acute subdural hematoma (with possible herniation syndromes) – 0.067,

5. history of kidney disease – 0.059,
6. history of diabetes mellitus – 0.058,
7. history of liver disease – 0.053,
8. presence of cerebral edema – 0.051,
9. neurological grade – 0.047,
10. history of hospital-acquired infections – 0.041,
11. thickness of subarachnoid hemorrhage – 0.037,
12. history of heart disease – 0.027,
13. presence of seizures requiring antiepileptic medications – 0.027,
14. presence of intraventricular hemorrhage – 0.026,
15. presence of intracerebral hemorrhage – 0.024,
16. presence of stroke – 0.021,
17. aneurysm location – 0.020,
18. aneurysm clipping – 0.020,
19. aneurysm coiling – 0.020,
20. history of lung disease – 0.019,
21. aneurysm size – 0.019,
22. sex – 0.013,
23. blood thinner use – 0.013,
24. presence of hypertension – 0.009, and
25. presence of delayed strokes – 0.008.

Discussion

Comparison of the artificial neural network models generated from the Tirilazad and Kurashiki Central Hospital aneurysmal subarachnoid hemorrhage databases yields several novel observations. Exploratory analyses reveal the complexity of brain-body interactions in influencing outcome in those with ruptured cerebral aneurysms. Our contemporary cohort from Kurashiki, Japan demonstrates:

1. patient management advances in the past two decades (namely, aneurysm securing techniques and vasospasm treatments, as these variables do not make significant contributions to patient outcomes in the contemporary cohort),
2. age and co-morbid burden differences between the two cohorts (average age of Tirilazad population was 52 years, versus 64 years for Kurashiki cohort),
3. differences in physiologic responses to aneurysmal subarachnoid hemorrhage and treatment based on genetics (Tirilazad databases did not capture patient populations from the East), and
4. importance of brain-body interactions in influencing outcomes in both cohorts (for disease entities such as kidney, liver, diabetes, which may predispose to presence of brain swelling on presentation).

Other variables, not directly measured, which also influence clinical outcomes in aneurysmal subarachnoid hemorrhage patients include:

1. disrupted cerebral autoregulation contributing to both ischemia and cerebral edema after subarachnoid hemorrhage,
2. biochemical markers of brain injury predisposing to cortical spreading depression,
3. cellular markers demonstrating physiologic dysfunction (such as mitochondrial dysfunction as reflected by imbalance between oxygen supply and consumption),
4. genetic factors affecting outcome (such as inheritance of genes making patients more prone to microthrombotic events in the cerebral microvasculature disrupting cerebral blood flow),

5. multiple drug-drug interactions, especially in the elderly aneurysmal subarachnoid hemorrhage patient population with multiple pre-existing comorbidities,
6. multi-organ system dysfunctions, including interactions between the central nervous system, and hematologic, gastrointestinal (including liver and splenic), neuro-endocrinologic and metabolic homeostasis, and
7. variables known to affect clinical outcome that were not captured in the Kurashiki Central Hospital database, including patient weight, smoking and alcohol consumption.

Exploratory analyses using artificial neural networks reveal the complexity of brain-body interactions in aneurysmal subarachnoid hemorrhage, as manifestations of dysfunctions of the autonomic nervous system. In the following points and paragraphs, we provide more insight on such pathophysiologic mechanisms, in addition to those found in previous sections of this work.

1. different levels of the nervous system contribute to various autonomic functions: (1) forebrain, hypothalamic and limbic control of autonomic and endocrine responses for cardiovascular and endocrinologic homeostasis (for example, prefrontal cortex and right insular region controlling heart rate variability, heart rhythm and blood pressure), (2) brainstem (pontomedullary level) control of cardiovascular, respiratory and autonomic signal integration, (3) altered central and spinal autonomic responses manifesting as changes in bladder detrusor activity and gastrointestinal motility, particularly in those with underlying predisposing conditions such as diabetic neuropathy.
2. interplay between the sympathetic and parasympathetic nervous system innervation of cerebral blood vessels. The parasympathetic system includes pterygopalatine ganglion

(vasoactive intestinal peptide), otic ganglion (peptide histidine methionine), and carotid ganglion (nitric oxide). Cholinergic innervation is most dense at cerebral vessel branching points, most noted in pial vessels. Sympathetic innervation includes the superior cervical ganglion (norepinephrine, neuropeptide Y) with neurons synapses in the loop from the hypothalamus, intermediolateral cell column of the spinal cord, to superior cervical ganglion. Sympathetic nerve terminals are found in the outer media layer of cerebral vessels, most dense in the anterior circulation, with autoregulatory and chemical contributions from both the superior cervical ganglion and pontine locus ceruleus. Finally, sensory innervation is noted with transmitters from the trigeminovascular system (substance P, calcitonin gene related peptide, neurokinin A). Vasodilatory, anti-inflammatory and parasympathetic nitric oxide mediated effects of milrinone can be used to overcome primary and secondary injury cascade related sequelae predisposing to both microvasculature and macrovasculature vasospasm.

3. increased basal sympathetic discharges and disrupted autoregulation of sympathetic outflow seen in conditions including hypertension, renal insufficiency, heart failure and liver dysfunction causing a vicious cycle of increased catecholamine release, increased activation of renin-angiotensin-aldosterone system, shunting of blood from venous to arterial system, with congestion in both systems, predisposing to edema formation and hemorrhage. Targeting the many autonomic receptors in both vasculature and end organs such as the heart, liver, kidney and spleen, one can aim to investigate for different ways of better controlling autonomic nervous system responses in both states of health and disease.

Conclusion

Exploratory analyses using artificial neural networks point to the complexity of the brain-body interface in influencing outcomes in patients with cerebrovascular disorders.

Section Six

Conclusion

Benjamin W. Y. Lo [*]
Departments of Neurosurgery,
Neurology and Critical Care Medicine,
Montreal Neurological Institute and Hospital,
McGill University, Montreal, Canada

Aneurysmal SAH affects the cardiopulmonary system with subsequent neuro-cardio-endocrinological responses as part of the secondary injury cascade in response to the primary ictus of aneurysmal SAH. Sympathetic activation of the cardiovascular system in aneurysmal SAH not only triggers the release of atrial and brain natriuretic peptide, it can also lead to increased pulmonary venous pressures and permeability causing hydrostatic pulmonary edema. Natriuretic states can herald the onset or worsening of clinical

[*] Corresponding Author Email: benjamin.lo@mcgill.ca.

vasospasm as the renin-angiotensin-aldosterone system is activated in a delayed manner.

A systematic review and critical appraisal of methodologic quality of existing studies that derive clinical predictor tools and clinical predictors used to determine outcome prognosis in patients with aneurysmal SAH reveals that the most frequently retained significant clinical prognostic factors for long-term neurologic outcome prediction include age and neurological grade. Yet, systematic reviews for clinical prognostic factors and clinical prediction tools in aneurysmal SAH have a number of methodological challenges. Several factors should be taken into account when determining the effect sizes of individual prognostic factors, including within and between study patient heterogeneity, variations in treatment, patient referral biases and prognostic viewpoints across different cultures.

Brain-body associations are essential in influencing outcome in patients with ruptured brain aneurysms (Figure 6.1).

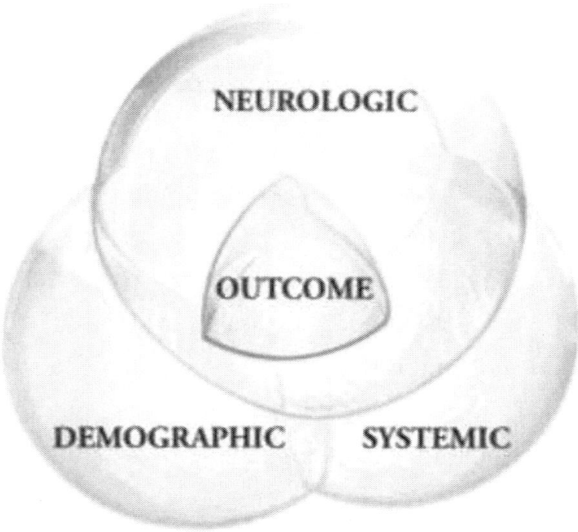

Figure 6.1. Diagram shows interlocking thematic clusters of prognostic risk factors in aneurysmal subarachnoid hemorrhage.

Aneurysmal SAH patients with history of hypertension and liver disease are predisposed to poor neurological outcome if they have concomitant cerebral edema. These patients have impaired cerebral autoregulation with disrupted blood brain barriers and altered collateral circulations. In addition, the epileptic aneurysmal SAH patient who develops post admission fever and myocardial infarction are predisposed to poor neurological outcome. Fevers increase cerebral metabolic rate and exacerbate secondary injury, including vasospasm-induced delayed strokes. Repetitive synchronized autonomic sympathetic discharges lead to cardiac ischemia and structural damage of the myocardium.

Aneurysmal subarachnoid hemorrhage prognosis models can be illustrated with the following four scenarios:

1. patient's initial and final clinical outcome prognosis designated as good (Figure 6.2).

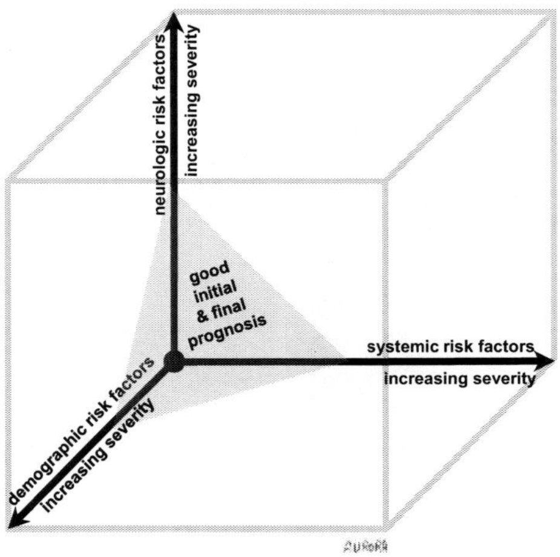

Figure 6.2. Zone of good initial and final prognosis.

2. patient's initial and final clinical outcome prognosis designated as poor (Figure 6.3).

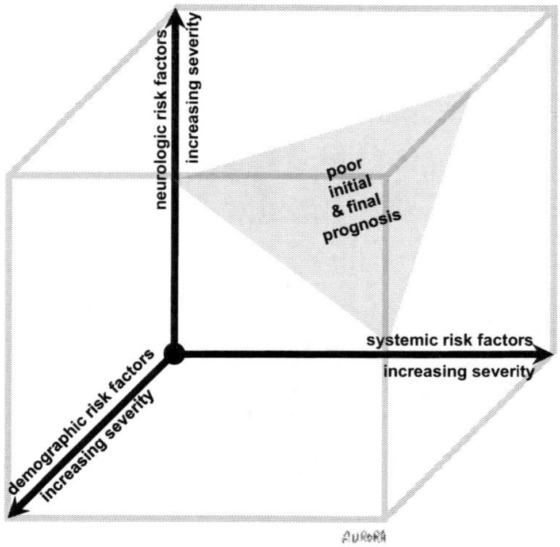

Figure 6.3. Zone of poor initial and final prognosis.

3. patient's initial prognosis designated as poor, but clinically improves over time with treatment. Hence, the final prognosis is also improved (Figure 6.4).

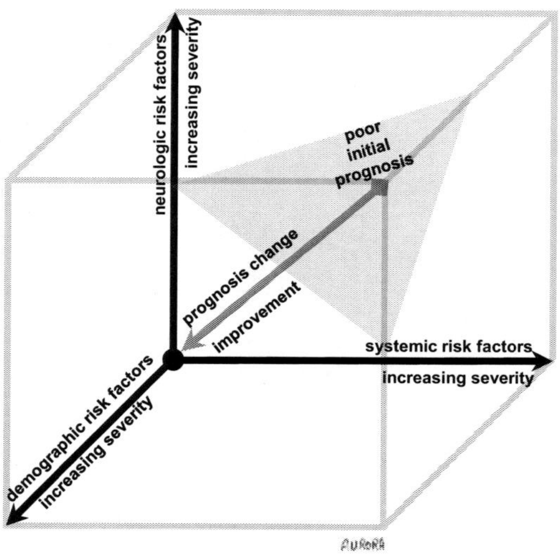

Figure 6.4. Poor initial prognosis with clinical improvement over time.

4. patient's initial prognosis designated as good, but clinically deteriorates over time with treatment. Hence, the final prognosis is designated as poor (Figure 6.5)

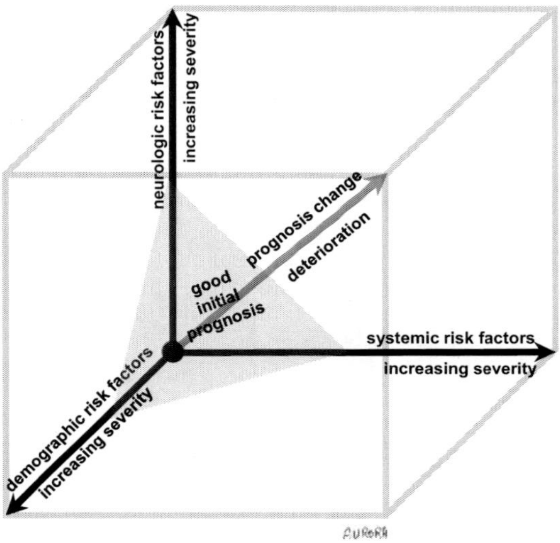

Figure 6.5. Good initial prognosis with clinical deterioration over time.

Classification and regression tree technique can be used to create decision-making algorithms for aneurysmal SAH patients, tools which can aid bedside prognostication and clinical treatment decision-making. Our decision tree revealed seven prognostic subgroups with important explanatory nodes including neurological grade, age, post admission fever and post admission stroke. In addition, post admission fever is demonstrated to be associated with increased odds of post admission strokes, including vasospasm-induced cerebral ischemia.

Future Directions

Given the rapid advances in diagnosis and treatment of aneurysmal SAH, future studies aim to generalize brain-body associations as well as decision-making algorithm to other aneurysmal SAH patient populations. Additional studies on pathophysiologic mechanisms of brain-body interactions in aneurysmal SAH will further shed light on how the brain communicates with other body systems under states of physiologic stress. Furthermore, investigations will be performed to see whether these associations in an altered brain-body interface are observed in patients with other acute cerebrovascular disorders, including ischemic and hemorrhage strokes.

Index

A

a priori hypotheses, 71, 72
accelerated gastric emptying, 30
activation function, 111, 115
acute lung injury, 46, 58, 102
acute myocardial infarction, 22
acute subdural hematoma, 70, 93, 110, 115
adrenal-hypothalamic cortisol axis, 20
adrenergic neurons, 8
afferent pulmonary vagal fibers, 10
Africa, 64, 86
age, 3, 21, 42, 44, 45, 46, 47, 48, 49, 50, 51, 64, 67, 69, 71, 73, 74, 75, 76, 77, 78, 91, 92, 95, 98, 100, 102, 107, 109, 113, 115, 117, 122, 125
alcohol, 46, 58, 118
aldosterone, 18, 28
ammonia, 81
amygdala, 6
anaerobic metabolism, 8
anemia, 30
aneurysm, xiv, 2, 3, 4, 5, 7, 11, 22, 28, 30, 42, 44, 45, 46, 47, 48, 49, 50, 51, 59, 60, 65, 66, 67, 68, 70, 74, 84, 85, 87, 88, 91, 93, 104, 108, 110, 113, 116, 117
aneurysm clipping, 47, 48, 49, 66, 70, 93, 110, 116
aneurysm coiling, 47, 48, 49, 66, 67, 116
aneurysm location, 49, 50, 51, 65, 70, 93, 110, 116
aneurysm size, 42, 44, 45, 46, 48, 49, 50, 68, 70, 74, 91, 93, 108, 110, 113, 116
aneurysm trapping with bypass, 66
aneurysmal rupture, 3, 18, 19, 20, 27, 37, 43, 65, 82, 95
aneurysmal subarachnoid hemorrhage, i, iii, v, vi, vii, xiii, 1, 2, 3, 11, 12, 13, 14, 17, 26, 27, 28, 29, 30, 32, 33, 35, 37, 39, 41, 57, 58, 59, 60, 61, 62, 63, 65, 83, 84, 85, 86, 88, 89, 95, 96, 97, 98, 99, 102, 103, 104, 105, 107, 111, 114, 116, 117, 118, 122, 123
angina, 68, 108, 113
angiographic vasospasm, 48, 68, 91, 108, 113

angiotensin converting enzyme inhibitor, 19
angiotensin II, 18, 80
angiotensin-converting enzyme inhibitors, 17, 31
anterior cingulate gyrus, 6
anterior cingulum, 81
anterior circulation aneurysms, 49
anticoagulant, 69, 92, 109
anticonvulsant use, 50
antiepileptic medications, 68, 74, 91, 93, 108, 116
anti-inflammatory, 101, 119
antioxidant, 66
antiplatelet, 69, 92, 109
anxiety disorder, 48
aorta, 9, 10
aortic arch, 6, 8, 82
aortic arch and carotid bodies, 6
aortic vessels, 8
area postrema, 6
arrhythmia, 22, 48
arrthymias, 79, 82
arterial baroceptors, 8
arterial baroreceptors, 6, 8
arterial blood gases, 23
arterio-alveolar gradient, 45
arteriosclerosis, 3
arteriovenous malformations, 21, 59
artificial neural networks, viii, 87, 106, 111, 112, 114, 118, 120
ascertainment bias, 41, 52
ascertainment of exposure, 41
ascorbic acid, 66
astrocytes, 81
ataxic breathing, 63
atherosclerotic changes, 71
atrial natriuretic peptide, 18, 19, 22, 23, 27
atrioventricular conduction, 9
Australia, 64, 85, 86
autonomic control, 10, 63
autonomic nervous control, 63
autonomic nervous system, vii, 6, 7, 8, 9, 118, 119
autonomic stimulation, 79
autonomic visceral afferents, 6
autoregulation, 81, 117, 119, 123

B

balloon angioplasty, 69, 109
baroreceptor sensitivity, 9, 82
baroreceptors, 8, 9, 10, 63
baroreflex, 9, 82
baroreflex neural network, 82
basal ganglia, 81
basal sympathetic discharges, 119
bedside prognostication, 90, 125
Beng-Teck Taw, Benedict, iii, xiii
beta adrenergic, 80
beta blockers, 82
bias, 41, 52, 53, 54, 55
bicarbonate, 45
binary logistic regression, 62, 71, 76, 77
binary logistic regression model, 71, 76, 77
bladder detrusor, 118
blinding, 52, 53, 54, 55
blood brain barriers, 30, 81, 123
blood carbon dioxide level, 8
blood clot thickness, 42, 44
blood oxygen, 8, 63
blood oxygen level, 8
blood pressure, 8, 9, 28, 51, 63, 65, 81, 82, 118
blood thinner, 69, 92, 109, 116
blood vessel constriction, 9
blood vessel endothelium, 28
blood vessel stretch, 9
blood-brain barrier disruption, 82, 101

boot-strapping, 37
brain natriuretic peptide, 18, 19, 22, 26, 28, 121
brain swelling, 3, 5, 37, 70, 77, 93, 110, 117
brain-body associations, vii, 11, 12, 13, 14, 15, 17, 18, 19, 22, 25, 27, 28, 31, 33, 44, 56, 62, 78, 86, 101, 102, 103, 122, 125
brain-body interactions, i, iii, vii, xi, 5, 6, 29, 32, 62, 71, 83, 86, 106, 107, 116, 117, 118, 126
brain-body interface, v, vi, viii, 1, 6, 10, 26, 32, 61, 63, 86, 102, 105, 120, 126
brain-gastrointestinal, 31
brain-immune systems, 31
brainstem, 6, 8, 9, 10, 23, 63, 118
brainstem chemoreceptors, 63
brainstem dysfunction, 23

C

C statistic, 111
calcitonin gene related peptide, 119
calcium, 5, 64
calcium channel blockers, 64
calibration, 43
candidate predictors, 41, 91
carbon dioxide, 8, 10, 63
cardiac, 8, 9, 10, 17, 18, 21, 22, 23, 24, 26, 28, 33, 47, 59, 64, 79, 85, 123
cardiac arrthymias, 64
cardiac asystole, 80
cardiac atrium, 10, 27
cardiac beta receptor hyperactivation, 26
cardiac contractility, 9, 27
cardiac ejection fraction, 26
cardiac enzyme elevation, 21
cardiac enzymes, 18, 19, 21
cardiac function index, 24
cardiac index, 22
cardiac ischemia, 79, 123
cardiac output, 9
cardiac stunning, 26
cardiac sympathetic discharges, 79
cardiac system, 17
cardiac troponin, 21, 22, 33, 47
cardiac troponin elevation, 21, 22, 33
cardiac ventricle, 26
cardiopulmonary, 12, 20, 21, 22, 23, 24, 28, 33, 121
cardiovascular disease, 64
cardiovascular instability, 45
carotid, 8, 9, 63, 82, 119
carotid arteries, 9
carotid ganglion, 119
carotid sinus, 8, 63, 82
carotid sinus baroreceptors, 63
CART, 52, 91, 104
CART decision trees, 91
catecholamine, 26, 28, 30, 63, 80, 119
catecholamine release, 26, 63, 119
catecholamine surges, 28
center cluster effects, 44
central (hypothalamic) damage, 30
central neurological injury, 101
central venous pressures, 24
cerebral blood flow, 81, 87, 117
cerebral cortex, 6, 9
cerebral dysautoregulation, 81
cerebral edema, 26, 30, 48, 66, 68, 73, 74, 75, 76, 78, 80, 81, 91, 101, 108, 113, 116, 117, 123
cerebral hyperemia, 81
cerebral infarction, 48, 50, 59, 82, 85
cerebral metabolic rates, 30, 72
cerebral perfusion deficits, 82
cerebral perfusion pressure, 46
cerebral surveillance, 82
cerebral vascular malformations, 3

cerebral vasospasm, 47, 59, 64, 85, 103
cerebrospinal fluid concentrations, 10
cervical and thoracic spinal cord, 10
chemoreceptors, 8, 63
chest radiograph, 19, 20, 21, 22, 23
chi-square analyses, 71, 94
cholinergic innervation, 119
chronic hydrocephalus, 70, 93, 110
chronic hypertensive, 81
chronotrophy, 8
circumventricular organ, 6
cisternal and ventricular blood, 51
cisternal flush, 66
classification accuracy, 94, 95
classification and regression tree analysis, viii, 32, 86, 90, 94
classification trees, 94, 100
clinical decision-making, 90, 100
clinical grade (WFNS, Hunt and Hess), 45
clinical opinion and judgment, 36, 90
clinical prediction tools, 36, 38, 39, 42, 43, 44, 56, 100, 103, 122
clinical predictor tools, vii, 36, 37, 122
clinical predictors, vii, 36, 37, 43, 122
clinical prognostic decision-making tools, viii
clinical prognostic factors, 42, 43, 100, 111, 122
clinical vasospasm, 18, 28, 122
clot thickness, 45, 50
coagulation, 30
coding and reproducibility, 36
cohort studies, 44, 56
collateral circulations, 82, 123
confounding, 42, 52, 53, 54, 55
confusion, 68, 108
congestive heart failure, 22, 48, 64
consciousness, 45, 51
contractile properties, 72
contraction band necrosis, 26
coronary artery disease, 48, 79
coronary blood flow, 26
cortical epileptiform activity, 79
cortical spreading depression, 82, 101, 117
corticosteroids, 31, 64
cortisol, 19, 30, 72
cortisol levels, 19, 72
cough, 29
counter-regulatory, 8, 63
counter-regulatory feedback, 8, 63
cranial nerve palsy, 68, 108
craniosacral (parasympathetic) levels, 6
creatinine clearance, 18
C-statistic, 52, 53, 54
Cushing reflex, 8
cytotoxic osmoregulatory mechanisms, 81

D

data splitting, 37
databases, vii, 12, 38, 42, 67, 76, 77, 78, 83, 91, 93, 107, 116
daughter nodes, 90
death, 21, 26, 49, 50, 59, 65, 69, 70, 81, 92, 93, 94, 100, 109, 111
decision tree, 90, 93, 94, 125
decompensated heart failure, 72
decompression, 66
decompressive craniectomy, 101
decreased nitric oxide, 5, 80
deep coma, 68, 108
deep venous thrombosis, 29
delayed cerebral ischemia, 21, 46
delayed stroke, 5, 26, 28, 30, 37, 70, 73, 74, 76, 79, 93, 101, 102, 110, 116, 123
demographic risk factors, 67, 69, 92, 107, 109
depression, 48
dexamethasone, 19, 20

diabetes, 48, 68, 69, 71, 73, 74, 75, 76, 84, 92, 108, 109, 113, 116, 117
diabetes mellitus, 68, 69, 84, 92, 108, 109, 113, 116
diagnostic CT angiograms, 66
diagnostic tests, 11, 12, 14, 15, 16, 18, 19, 20, 21, 22, 23
diaphragm, 10
diastolic blood pressure, 9, 67, 107, 113
diencephalon, 6
diffuse vasospasm, 49
discrimination, 43, 111
diuretic, 17, 19, 28
diversion, 70, 93, 110
dorsal motor nucleus of vagus, 8
dromotropy, 8
drug-drug interactions, 30, 79, 101, 118

E

early onset fevers, 30, 79
early-onset cerebral edema, 31
echocardiogram, 20, 21
echocardiograph, 22
echocardiography, 18
edema formation, 27, 119
elastic lamina, 2
elasticity, 71
electrocardiogram, 18, 19, 20, 21
electrocardiograph, 22
electrolyte and fluid balance, 17
endocrine diseases, 19
endocrine response, 17, 18, 24, 31, 32, 118
endocrine system, 17, 63
endocrinological functions, 10
endothelial damage, 71
endothelial function, 30
endothelial hypertrophy, 72
endothelial relaxation, 80
endothelin, 5, 19, 80
endothelin I, 80
endothelin-1, 5
endovascular techniques, 12, 66
epilepsy, xv, 79, 83, 84, 85, 87
epinephrine, 19
error functions, 107
Europe, 64, 85, 86
euvolemia, 17, 18
exclusion criteria, 13, 15, 19, 20, 21, 22, 23, 39, 41
exploratory analyses, vi, viii, 105, 106, 116, 118, 120
external validation techniques, 37
extravascular lung water index, 22, 24, 26
extravascular lung water indices, 23

F

fasudil, 66
fevers, 5, 30, 37, 50, 68, 72, 73, 74, 75, 76, 77, 79, 85, 87, 88, 91, 94, 95, 98, 100, 101, 102, 108, 113, 123, 125
fibrinolysis, 30
fibrinolytic markers, 30
Fisher grade, 47, 49, 50, 51
follow-up, 36, 41, 43
free radical production, 30
free radical scavenger, 64
Fukuda, Hitoshi, iii, v, vi, ix, xiii, 1, 12, 35, 38, 61, 89, 105
functional dependence, 69, 70, 92, 93, 94, 109, 111
functional independence, 69, 70, 92, 93, 109, 111

G

gastric ulcers, 30

gastrointestinal, 10, 13, 17, 30, 118
gastrointestinal autonomic nervous system, 10
gastrointestinal motility, 30, 118
gastrointestinal system, 17
genetics, 117
Gini index splitting rule, 93
Glasgow coma score, 45
Glasgow outcome scale, 45, 49, 50
Glasgow outcome score, 45, 46, 47, 51, 65, 69, 92, 109, 112, 114
global ejection fraction, 24
global end diastolic volume index, 24
glomerular filtration rate, 18
glossopharyngeal and vagus nerves, 8
glucose, 45, 47, 51
glutamate, 81
good recovery, 65
gut motility, 10

H

headaches, 68, 108
health-related quality of life, 5, 37
heart disease, 69, 77, 92, 109, 116
heart failure, 72, 119
heart rate, 8, 9, 32, 79, 80, 82, 85, 118
heart rate oscillations, 9
heart rate variability, 9, 32, 79, 80, 82, 85, 118
hematologic, 3, 13, 118
hematologic dyscrasias, 3
hemiparesis, 68, 108
hemodynamic factors, 47
hemoglobin, 48, 59
hepatic, 19, 68, 72, 76, 78, 81, 87, 108, 113
hepatic disease, 68, 76, 78, 108, 113
hepatic dysfunction, 72
hepatic encephalopathy, 81
heterogeneity, 65
hidden layer, 111, 115
high dimensionality, 91
high frequency power, 9
high order interactions, 91
Hijdra scale, 70, 93, 110
holdout sample, 111, 115
homeostasis, 10, 63, 85, 118
Hosmer-Lemeshow, 52, 54
hospital-acquired infections, 69, 92, 110, 116
humoral, 6
Hunt and Hess, 46, 47, 48, 49, 51, 68, 76, 91, 94, 95, 108
hydrocephalus, 5, 37, 48, 51, 68, 75, 77, 108, 114, 115
hydrogen ions, 8, 10
hydrostatic pressures, 27, 81
hydrostatic pulmonary edema, 27, 29, 63, 121
hypercatabolic, 30
hypercontraction, 26
hyperglycemia, 45, 48, 59, 103
hypertension, 3, 45, 47, 48, 49, 50, 68, 69, 71, 73, 74, 75, 76, 78, 80, 81, 87, 91, 92, 108, 109, 114, 116, 119, 123
hypertensive therapy, 21
hyperventilation, 63
hypervolemia, 50
hypotension, 21, 26
hypothalamic, 6, 10, 63, 118
hypothalamic paraventricular nucleus, 6
hypothalamic-pituitary axis, 10, 63
hypothalamus, 6, 79, 119
hypoxia, 45

I

IBM SPSS, 70, 91, 107, 111, 112, 114, 115

ictal tachycardia, 79
immobility, 29
immune, 13, 17, 29
immune and hematologic systems, 17
immune systems, 29
inappropriate predictor models, 39, 41
inclusion and exclusion criteria, 14, 15, 36, 40, 42
increased preload, 27, 29
infections, 29, 30, 79
infectious mycotic aneurysms, 64
inflammatory cell migration, 30
inflammatory cytokines, 30, 79
inotropic and vasopressor support, 31
inotropic effects, 8
inotropic vasodilator, 101
inotropy, 8
inspiratory cycle, 9
insula, 6
insular region, 118
insulin, 71, 80
insulin resistance, 71
interactions, vii, 26, 28, 44, 56, 62, 67, 71, 78, 79, 101, 103, 118
intercostal muscles, 10
intermediolateral cell column, 119
intermediolateral spinal cord, 6
internal validation techniques, 36
internodal connection, 106
interrater reliability, 39
Interrater reliability, 13
intestinal motility, 30
intracerebral hemorrhage, vii, 3, 8, 46, 48, 51, 68, 70, 75, 91, 93, 108, 110, 116
intracranial pressure, 3, 8, 46, 51, 57, 60, 101
intraparenchymal hematoma, 49
intrathoracic blood volume index, 22
intrathoracic blood volume indices, 23
intraventricular blood, 49
intraventricular hemorrhage, 26, 45, 46, 50, 51, 68, 70, 74, 75, 91, 93, 108, 110, 113, 116
ischemic injury, 30
ischemic stroke, vii

K

kappa statistic, 13, 39
Karnofsky scale, 45
Kasuya, Hidetoshi, iii, vi, xiv, 105
kidney disease, 69, 77, 92, 109, 116
kidney function, 30
Koyanagi, Masaomi, iii, v, vi, xiii, 1, 61, 89, 105
Kurashiki Central Hospital, ix, 62, 65, 67, 69, 76, 77, 90, 91, 92, 99, 100, 106, 107, 109, 114, 116, 118
Kyoto University, xiii, 62, 90, 106

L

lactic acid, 4
late onset fevers, 30, 79, 101
latent (unobservable) variables, 56, 106, 111, 115
left ventricular ejection fraction, 47
leukocytosis, 48
Levine, Mitchell A. H., iii, v, vi, xv, 1, 35, 61, 89, 105
limbic, 6, 10, 63, 118
limbic cortex, 6
limbic system, 10
liver disease, 69, 72, 73, 74, 75, 76, 80, 81, 87, 92, 109, 116, 123
liver dysfunction, 72, 81, 119
Lo, Aurora W. M., iii, xiv
Lo, Benjamin W. Y., v, vi, xi, 1, 35, 61, 89, 105, 121

local paracrine pathways, 11
locus ceruleus, 6
long-term disability, 5, 37
loss of consciousness, 26
low frequency component, 79
low frequency power, 9, 82
lung disease, 69, 92, 109, 116
lung inflation and deflation, 9, 10
lungs, 9
luxury perfusion, 81

M

mathematical methods, 41
mathematical models, 36
mean arterial pressure, 45, 49
mechanical ventilation, 47
media layer, 119
medical history, 48
medulla, 6, 10
medullary chemoreceptors, 10
medullary raphe, 6
mesial temporal lobe seizures, 79
metabolic acidosis, 45
methodologic quality, vii, 13, 14, 24, 36, 37, 39, 40, 42, 43, 122
methodologic quality assessment, 13, 14, 39, 40
microthrombi formation, 82, 101
microthrombotic events, 117
microvasuclar constriction, 82
midbrain, 6
middle cerebral artery flow velocity, 51
migraines, 68, 108, 113
milrinone, 66, 85, 101, 119
mitochondrial dysfunction, 117
model classification, 111
model performance, 52, 53
moderate disability, 65
modified Fisher score, 70, 93, 110
morbidity, 21, 22, 33, 72, 79
moribund, 68, 108
mortality, 3, 22, 32, 46, 48, 49, 51, 58, 72, 78, 103
multi-organ involvement, 18, 19
multivariable, 52, 53, 54, 55, 71, 76, 77, 100
multivariable analyses, 71
myocardial infarction, 5, 26, 37, 48, 64, 68, 72, 73, 74, 75, 76, 78, 79, 85, 91, 108, 113, 123

N

natriuretic peptides, 22, 23, 27, 30, 63
nerve impulse, 9
network architecture, 111, 115
neuro-cardio-endocrine response, 18
neuro-cardio-endocrine systems, 28
neurocritical care, xi, 12, 33, 58, 66, 88, 101
neuroendocrine, 12, 19, 83
neurogenic pulmonary edema, 20, 21, 23, 24, 32, 80
neurohumoral activation, 30
neurokinin A, 119
neurologic and functional outcomes, viii
neurological grade, 26, 42, 44, 46, 49, 50, 65, 68, 70, 72, 73, 76, 77, 78, 92, 94, 95, 98, 100, 102, 108, 110, 113, 116, 122, 125
neuronal excitability, 79
neuronal hypoxic damage, 30
neuronal ischemic threshold, 30
neuronal swelling, 81
neuropeptide Y, 119
New Zealand, 64, 85, 86
nimodipine, 64

Nishimura, Yusuke, iii, xiv
nitric oxide, 119
nitrogen loss, 30
node, 90, 94, 95
non-linear, 91, 106
norepinephrine, 19, 119
North America, 3, 37, 64, 65, 84, 85
nosocomial infections, 101
nucleus ambiguus, 8
nucleus of the solitary tract, 6
nucleus tractus solitarius, 6, 8

O

obesity, 3, 48
occipital lobes, 81
oncotic pressures, 27
optimization processes, 107
organ dysfunction, 14, 15, 33
otic ganglion, 119
outcome, vii, 13, 14, 15, 21, 32, 33, 36, 37, 38, 39, 41, 42, 43, 44, 45, 46, 47, 48, 49, 50, 51, 56, 57, 58, 59, 60, 62, 65, 67, 69, 70, 71, 72, 73, 74, 75, 77, 78, 79, 80, 81, 82, 83, 84, 85, 86, 87, 88, 91, 92, 93, 94, 95, 98, 100, 101, 102, 103, 104, 107, 109, 111, 116, 117, 118, 122, 123
outcome assessments, 41, 43
overfitting, 90, 94
oxygen, 4, 8, 10, 30, 117
oxygen tension, 10

P

pacemaker cells, 10, 63
pain stimulus, 8
parabrachial nucleus, 6
parasympathetic, 9, 79, 80, 118
parasympathetic activity, 79, 80
parasympathetic nervous activity, 9
parasympathetic tone, 9
paravertebral chain, 26
parent artery occlusion, 66
pathophysiologic mechanisms, v, vii, 1, 11, 12, 13, 14, 15, 17, 22, 27, 28, 31, 33, 44, 86, 102, 103, 118, 126
patient heterogeneity, 43, 122
patient inclusion, 13, 15, 39, 41
patient population, 14, 24, 41, 44, 78, 83, 94, 117, 118, 126
patient recruitment, 36
patient selection, 18, 20, 21, 23, 24, 43
peptide histidine methionine, 119
periaqueductal gray matter, 6
peripheral arterioles, 26
peripheral vascular resistance, 9
permeability, 27, 81, 121
persistent vegetative state, 65, 69, 92, 94, 109
pH levels, 63
physical, neurocognitive and psychological impairment, 5, 37
physiologic dysfunction, 21, 117
physiological derangements, 26
physiological stress, 5, 6, 72
pial vessels, 119
PiCCO system, 22
placebo, 64, 65
plasma aldosterone, 19
plasma electrolytes, 6
plasma proteins, 81
plasma sodium levels, 19, 23, 28
plasma vasopressin levels, 19
pneumonia, 29
pneumotaxic neurons, 10
pons, 6, 10
pontine locus ceruleus, 119
posterior cerebral circulation, 81
posterior circulation aneurysms, 20, 49

potential confounding variables, 41, 43
prediction tools, 36, 43, 44
predictor variables, 36, 43, 44
predictors, 36, 41, 44, 56, 59, 103
prefrontal cortex, 118
pregnant, 64
primary injury, 3, 24
primary neurological injury, 37
prognosis, vii, 36, 37, 39, 44, 56, 59, 78, 82, 122, 123, 124, 125
prognostic decision-making algorithms, vi, 89
prognostic factors, v, viii, 35, 38, 39, 42, 43, 44, 56, 60, 69, 71, 78, 83, 92, 102, 103, 104, 106, 109, 122
programmed cell death, 5
pro-inflammatory cascade, 82, 101
prospective, vii, 11, 16, 17, 18, 22, 23, 25, 38, 39, 42, 52, 53, 54, 55
prospective and retrospective cohort studies, vii, 11, 38, 39
prospective cohort studies, 16, 42
pterygopalatine ganglion, 118
publication bias, 41
pulmonary, 5, 8, 10, 16, 17, 23, 26, 28, 29, 30, 31, 33, 37, 46, 48, 58, 63, 68, 79, 108, 114, 121
pulmonary arteries, 10
pulmonary artery thermodilution parameters, 16
pulmonary capillaries, 29
pulmonary capillary pressure, 29
pulmonary disease, 48
pulmonary edema, 5, 23, 26, 28, 31, 33, 37, 68, 108, 114
pulmonary embolism, 29, 30, 79
pulmonary hypertension, 28, 29
pulmonary infiltrates, 46, 58
pulmonary system, 17, 63
pulmonary vascular permeability, 27, 63
pulmonary vascular pressure, 27
pulmonary vasculature, 28
pulmonary venous pressures, 26, 121
pulsatility index, 51
pulse contour analysis, 12, 22, 23, 26
pyrogens, 79

Q

QRS complex, 9
QT prolongation, 20

R

randomization group, 49, 50
randomized controlled trials (RCTs), vii, 11, 38, 39, 42, 44, 56
randomized, double-blind, placebo-controlled trials, 64
reactive oxygen species, 5
rebleeding, 5, 20, 37, 45, 46, 51, 59, 70, 73, 74, 75, 77, 87, 93, 110
recall bias, 41, 43, 52, 53
receptors, 80, 82, 119
recruitment, 14, 15, 40
recursive partitioning, 90
red blood cell transfusions, 46
reference standard, 11, 15, 18, 19, 20, 21, 22, 23, 25
referral biases, 18, 20, 21, 23, 24, 41, 43, 44, 53, 55, 122
regional wall motion abnormalities, 47
renal, 12, 17, 19, 24, 28, 33, 48, 80, 119
renal disease, 48
renal insufficiency, 17, 119
renal systems, 19
renal tubules, 28
renin, 18, 19, 20, 27, 28, 31, 63, 80, 119, 122

renin levels, 19
renin-angiotensin-aldosterone system, 18, 20, 27, 28, 31, 63, 80, 119, 122
reproducibility, 41
resistance index, 51
respiration, 10, 63
respiratory sinus arrthymias, 9
respiratory suppression, 80
resuscitation, 27, 28
retrospective cohort studies, 42
retrospective study, 16
risk estimate, 94, 95
ROC curve, 111, 112, 115
rostral ventrolateral medulla, 8
RR interval, 9
RR interval changes, 9
ruptured brain aneurysms, 3, 11, 14, 15, 24, 31, 33, 56, 62, 65, 78, 86, 103, 122

S

salt balance, 18
sample size, 14, 18, 20, 21, 23, 24, 36, 41, 42, 44, 52, 53, 54, 55, 93
secondary injurious processes, 3, 5
secondary injury, 37, 79, 82, 101, 119, 121, 123
secretory functions, 11
seizures, 5, 37, 68, 73, 74, 75, 76, 77, 78, 79, 83, 84, 85, 87, 88, 91, 101, 108, 113, 116
selection and coding of data, 41
selection bias, 24, 41, 53, 55
selection criteria, 24, 25
sensory innervation, 119
sepsis, 46
severe disability, 65, 70, 93, 100, 111
sex, 45, 46, 47, 48, 49, 51, 64, 67, 69, 92, 107, 109, 114, 116
shunting, 70, 77, 93, 110, 119
shunting procedure, 70, 77, 93, 110
sick euthyroid syndrome, 72
sigmoid function, 111, 115
sinoatrial node, 8, 9
sinus node, 9, 79
smoking, 3, 47, 48, 118
sodium, 17, 23, 28, 30, 31, 48, 49, 63, 80
sodium and blood volume regulation, 17, 31
sodium and water balance, 28, 31
sodium level, 30, 48, 49
spinal reflexes, 10
split sample validation techniques, 90
spontaneous subarachnoid hemorrhage, 3
ST segment abnormalities, 20
standard error, 94, 95
starling forces, 29
statistical analysis, 65, 69, 109
statistical power, 41, 93
status epilepticus, 74
steroids, 17
stratification, 43, 52, 53, 54, 55
stroke, xi, 9, 30, 32, 33, 48, 57, 60, 62, 68, 70, 73, 76, 77, 78, 82, 83, 86, 90, 91, 93, 94, 95, 98, 100, 103, 104, 106, 108, 110, 113, 116, 125
stroke volume, 9, 30
study design, 14, 15, 24, 25, 40, 52, 53, 54, 55
study eligibility criteria, 11, 38
study power, 43, 44
study protocols, 15, 17, 19, 20, 21, 22, 23, 24, 42
stunned apical and mid-ventricular segments, 26
stunned myocardium, 31
stupor, 68, 108
subarachnoid clot thickness, 49

subarachnoid hemorrhage, vii, xiv, 3, 4, 17, 18, 20, 21, 22, 23, 25, 28, 31, 32, 33, 45, 49, 52, 57, 58, 59, 60, 68, 70, 83, 84, 85, 87, 93, 102, 108, 110, 113, 117
subdural hematoma, 51
substance P, 119
sudden cardiac death, 79, 82
superior cervical ganglion, 119
surgery, xiii, xiv, 66, 76, 77, 91
surgical clipping, 46, 64
sympathetic, 8, 9, 26, 63, 79, 80, 118, 119, 121, 123
sympathetic innervation, 119
sympathetic modulation, 9, 79
sympathetic nerve terminals, 119
sympathetic nervous system, 8, 26, 63, 80
sympathetic outflow, 80, 119
sympathetic overdrive, 79
sympathetic tone, 8
sympathetic vasomotor tone, 9
sympathovagal balance, 9, 82
symptomatic vasospasm, 46, 50, 66, 71, 82
synaptic weights, 106
synchronized neuronal activity, 79
synchronized time-locked manner, 79
systematic review, v, 11, 14, 15, 16, 33, 35, 36, 37, 38, 40, 43, 44, 56, 57, 58, 86, 88, 103, 122
systemic conditions, 73, 74
systemic inflammation, 51
systemic inflammatory states, 29, 30
systemic medical complications, 5, 37
systemic vascular resistance index, 22
systolic, 9, 21, 26, 50, 64, 67, 107, 113
systolic blood pressure, 9, 50, 65, 67, 107, 113

T

takotsubo-like cardiomyopathy, 26
tako-tsubo-like cardiomyopathy, 20, 21
tako-tsubo-like cardiomyopathy, 32
temperature control, 10
temperature on admission, 67, 107, 113
temperature sensitive ion channels, 79
testing dataset, 94, 95, 100
thickness of subarachnoid hemorrhage, 68, 108, 113, 116
thoracic paravertebral chain, 63
thoracolumbar (sympathetic), 6
thoracolumbar interomediolateral gray column of the spinal cord, 6
thromboembolic events, 101
thrombosis, 30
through muscle sympathetic nervous activity, 9
thyroid disease, 68, 72, 73, 108, 113
thyroid gland, 72
thyroid hormone, 72, 87
thyroxine production, 72
time to surgical treatment, 69, 109, 113
time to treatment, 64
Tirilazad, ix, 62, 64, 65, 67, 76, 77, 78, 88, 90, 91, 92, 94, 95, 96, 97, 98, 100, 106, 107, 111, 116, 117
Tirilazad database, ix, 62, 64, 76, 77, 78, 90, 92, 95, 96, 97, 98, 100, 106, 111, 117
training dataset, 94, 95, 100
training time, 111
transcranial Doppler, 18, 22, 60
transcranial Doppler ultrasound, 18
traumatic SAH, 21, 38, 39, 64
treatment protocols, 43
tree pruning, 94
trigeminovascular system, 119

troponin elevations, 26, 72
troponin release, 26
T-wave inversions, 20

U

uncontrolled hypertension, 64
univariate, 43, 52, 53, 54, 55, 56, 71, 91, 94
univariate and multivariable logistic regression analyses, 43, 56
univariate logistic regression analysis, 91
Upton, Adrian, iii, v, vi, xv, 1, 61, 89, 105
urinary sodium levels, 19
urokinase, 66

V

vagal activity, 8, 9
vagal withdrawal, 79
validation, 36, 41, 54, 55, 60, 100, 111
variable and outcome reporting, 39, 41
variables, 36, 41, 42, 44, 45, 46, 47, 48, 49, 50, 51, 57, 67, 69, 71, 76, 77, 91, 92, 94, 107, 109, 113, 115, 117, 118
variance, 93
variations, 43, 122
vascular baroreceptors, 63
vascular resistance vessels, 72
vasoactive intestinal peptide, 119
vasoconstrictors, 80
vasodilation, 29
vasodilatory, 8, 66, 119
vasodilatory effects, 8
vasogenic edema, 81
vasomotor area, 6
vasomotor regions, 8, 63
vasopressin, 18, 30
vasopressors, 20, 21, 26
vasospasm, xiv, 4, 5, 20, 21, 28, 37, 46, 50, 68, 69, 73, 74, 75, 84, 88, 91, 100, 101, 108, 109, 113, 117, 119, 122, 123, 125
vasospasm induced strokes, 37
veins, 9, 28
venous pressures, 63
ventilation, 9
ventilatory support, 31
ventricle, 10
ventricular dilation, 49
ventriculomegaly, 47
ventrolateral medulla, 6
vitamin C, 66

W

Wai-Man Lui, Matthew, vi, xiv, 105
Wan, Yee-Yin A., iii, xiv
water balance, 24
weight, 67, 107, 111, 113, 115, 118
WFNS grade, 46, 49, 50, 51, 100
withdrawals, 15, 24, 25
World Federation of Neurological Surgeons, 70, 92, 110